MORE PRAISE FOR *MY HOUSE IS KILLING ME!*

"With a sharp increase in the incidence of asthma, respiratory allergies, and other respiratory allergy symptoms, the need for clear information regarding environmental triggers is crucial. This guide identifies the sources of not only allergic but also irritant and toxic exposures in the home environment. This text, together with the author's extensive experience in evaluating homes for risks, provides patients and parents an invaluable resource to begin addressing some of their concerns and investigating possible causes of symptoms. Considering how much misinformation is provided in the lay press, it is reassuring to find a resource to which I can direct my patients for practical and reliable information!"

FRANK J. TWAROG
Associate Clinical Professor, Harvard Medical School

"I have had the opportunity to work with Jeff, and he is the 'real thing.' He has helped many of my patients. After reading *My House is Killing Me!* I am convinced that it is a must-read for patients with respiratory problems and the physicians who care for them. His book is also a must-read for anyone who owns a home or is about to purchase or renovate one."

RICHARD S. IRWIN, M.D.
University of Massachusetts Medical School

My House Is Killing Me!

JEFFREY C. MAY

My House Is Killing Me!

The Home Guide
for Families with
Allergies and
Asthma

FOREWORD BY
Jonathan M. Samet, M.D.

The Johns Hopkins University Press • Baltimore and London

616.97
MAY

Note to the reader: This book is not intended to provide medical or legal advice. The services of a competent professional should be obtained whenever medical, legal, or other specific advice is needed.

The Johns Hopkins University Press
2715 North Charles Street
Baltimore, Maryland 21218-4363
www.press.jhu.edu

Library of Congress Cataloging-in-Publication Data
May, Jeffrey C.
My house is killing me! : the home guide for families with allergies
and asthma / Jeffrey C. May ; foreword by Jonathan M. Samet.
p.   cm.
Includes bibliographical references and index.
ISBN 0-8018-6729-0 (hardcover : alk. paper) —
ISBN 0-8018-6730-4 (pbk. : alk. paper)
1. Allergy—Popular works. 2. Asthma—Popular works. 3. Indoor air
pollution—Popular works. I. Title.
RC 585 .M29 2001
616.97—dc21   00-012495

A catalog record for this book is available from the British Library.

CONTENTS

FOREWORD

My House Is Killing Me! may seem like a sensational title. But the stories related here by Jeffrey May, an experienced indoor air quality professional, clearly show the dangers of indoor allergens and other pollutants, particularly for those whom allergies make highly sensitive. In this book, Mr. May illustrates the potential dangers to health from indoor allergens, using a framework based on the different areas of the home. He draws on his vast experience, offering general lessons from the often dramatic stories of the people he has aided over his long career. Much as physicians cure sick persons, Mr. May and other indoor air quality professionals "cure" sick homes and buildings. Unless the *cause* of illnesses arising from indoor allergens or other pollutants is effectively addressed, medical treatments may be extended unnecessarily or may even be ineffective.

Even in the warmest and sunniest environments in the United States and other developed countries, we spend most of our time indoors. Hence the air we breathe and the pollutants in that air are often dominated by indoor sources. We accept many of these sources without much thought: humidifiers, pets, carpeting, and furnishings. But these features of our homes may be damaging to health, although this potential is often overlooked by affected people and the physicians who care for them. Professionals like Mr. May, informed physicians, and the community of researchers on indoor environments have identified and described exposure to pollutants in indoor environments and their potential effect on health. This work has made clear that indoor pollution sources, including those generating allergens, impair health and cause disease.

This book addresses the most severe effects, those making people so ill that they seek professional evaluations of their health and their homes. They are the tip of an iceberg, which has as its base a broad range of more subtle consequences for public health. To deal with the full problem of indoor air quality, we need to address the obvious health problems described in this book, and we also need to begin to avert indoor pollution problems through construction practices, codes, and other approaches.

This book will be informative for those who think their health problems may be caused by their homes. Such problems can be frustrating to affected persons and to their health care providers, who are often unaware that the quality of indoor environments is connected with health and disease. This book should be particularly valuable for the substantial number of people who have asthma and other allergic diseases. In fact the frequency of such diseases is rising, and indoor air problems are considered one possible explanation. Mr. May offers practical suggestions for diagnosing problems and for preventing them. Following his guidance, readers may find solutions.

For those who do not achieve a satisfactory resolution, what steps should they take next? Some health care providers may be able to provide informed diagnoses and treatment. Allergists and pulmonary physicians or specialists in occupational and environmental medicine are most likely to be "tuned in." Unfortunately there are many less knowledgeable health care providers, and both patients and providers may become frustrated trying to solve health problems that are based on an indoor air pollution source.

There are also many excellent indoor air quality professionals, like the author of this book. Some physicians work closely with such health professionals and will bring them in to help with specific cases if indicated. But some physicians may not know that there is a need for consultation. Therefore patients who are convinced that indoor pollution is a problem may want to consult an indoor air quality professional on their own. Finding the right knowledgeable professional may be hard, and it is important to avoid working with someone who may be uninformed. I suggest obtaining as much local guidance as possible: try to find "a gem" like Mr. May.

Fortunately he has written this book, which offers his solutions to a challenging set of problems.

Jonathan M. Samet, M.D.

ACKNOWLEDGMENTS

Because I learned something every time I completed an indoor air quality investigation, all the people who asked me to help them deserve my appreciation. There are some people, however, to whom I'd like to give special thanks:

Dr. Martha Stark, Kelley Leyba, Steve Goselin, and Barbara Craig, who gave me valuable feedback on my manuscript.

Jack Spengler and Jack McCarthy, who provided me with my first glimpse into the world of air quality and have continued to support my work.

John Knowles, who worked with me to produce the SEM images from my samples.

Dr. William Butler, without whom I couldn't have told the tale.

Connie May, who through her methodical approach taught me to sequence and clarify my muddled mess into this book.

My editor, Jacqueline Wehmueller, on whom I depended wholeheartedly and who never let me down.

Managing the Unseen

A young man who was having allergy symptoms in his house asked me to investigate. He greeted me with red eyes and a stuffy nose. At his side stood a large panting dog, its head nearly waist high. After I introduced myself, the first words out of the fellow's mouth were, "If you tell us that my wife's dog is causing my allergies, she's getting rid of *me*."

Another homeowner was experiencing allergy symptoms in every room of her house but one, a later addition. She left me a long phone message whose final words were, "My house is killing me!" I visited the home and found that the cartons and furniture stored in her basement were covered with mold. In the course of installing baseboard heating, a previous owner had removed the old furnace and most of the ducts. Unfortunately, the abandoned upstairs heat registers were still open to the basement. Basement air and mold spores floated up into every room in the house except the addition, which did not contain a register.

I have worked with hundreds of people who had problems with the quality of the air where they live and work, and I have witnessed how these problems affect their health—and their lives overall. Women and children seem to suffer the consequences of bad *indoor air quality* (IAQ) at about twice the rate men do. Often only one family member has become *sensitized* (is affected by allergens, chemicals, and other irritants), and it is common to find tension in such families. You may not be very sympathetic toward the suffering of others who have *allergies* (about one in four), *asthma* (about one in fourteen), or *chemical sensitivity,* an increased vulnerability to chemicals and other irritants found in the environment (more than one in twenty). It is important to realize, though, that these symptoms can afflict any one of us at any time. Even if you yourself have never (yet!) reacted negatively to an environment, you certainly know someone who has.

We accept as fact that some of us suffer from contact with poison ivy and others do not. One person will develop a small swelling at the site of a bee sting, but another may die within minutes. We think it perfectly normal that some of us are more sensitive to odors or can hear better than others. We recognize that some people have an acute sense of color and notice shades, while others do not see subtle hues. We don't all taste food the same way. This may be why certain foods—like spinach and olives—are either loathed or loved. A chemical called *phenylthiocarbamide* can be used to test a person's genetically determined sense of taste. For the test, you touch your tongue to a narrow strip of paper containing a minute amount of this chemical. Some people immediately grimace at the extremely bitter taste, while others find the paper tasteless.

We know we receive external information through our five senses, but few people realize that we inhale fragments of the outside world with every breath. In a way, the delicate surfaces of our lungs are in contact with the outside world just as our skin is. Why then do we tend to be suspicious when someone else seems to react to something in the air in a specific place and we don't? Perhaps if we could see the air and what it contains, just as we see colors and smell odors, we would be more understanding.

And what is in the air we breathe? Air contains many unseen *particulates,* or small particles: pollen, mold spores, bacteria, pet dander, insect parts, shed skin scales, fabric fibers, smoke, soot, and tire particles, to name a few. Air also contains invisible chemicals, some that we can smell, such as gasoline fumes, ammonia, and fragrances, and some that we cannot consciously sense because they are in concentrations below our "odor threshold." Ants use alarm *pheromones* (a chemical substance secreted by an animal that influences behavior) to muster their fellow soldiers. We see the troops battling on the pavement, but we don't sense their urgent, airborne messages. A female *Cecropia* moth secretes a sex pheromone that the male moth can detect miles downwind. (It is now believed that human physiology can also be affected by pheromones.

Science is recognizing what females have known all along: that women living or working together in groups will, within a few months, all menstruate at nearly the same time every month. Scientists believe that female sweat glands may emit a pheromone that causes this to happen.)

Even though we can't see air or most of what it contains, air is similar to water in that it is a fluid full of particles and chemicals. To keep fish happy and healthy in an aquarium, water must be aerated, cleaned by a filtering system, and circulated. No one would expect fish to survive in a closed jar of green, cloudy water. Likewise, indoor air that contains contaminates can make some people sick. The difference is that we cannot see the contamination in the air; if we could, bad air would look as murky as stagnant water and we would know we shouldn't breathe it in.

Like an aquarium, a house may be a closed environment, with the basement, the attic, and the rooms in which people live most of the time all interconnected by the air flowing throughout them, as well as by the components of the heating, ventilating, and air conditioning (HVAC) systems. Our activities indoors and the operation of the HVAC systems are "coupled." In a basement or crawl space, for example, operation of a heating or cooling system can lower the air pressure. This *depressurization* creates an airflow from the outside of a home to the inside. As a result, soil gases can be drawn through floor and foundation cracks and pipe openings, bringing moisture, odors, mold spores, or radon gas into the interior. At the same time as the basement is depressurized, the upstairs of a home may be pressurized, forcing moist indoor air into the walls or a cool attic and causing moisture to condense. In newer homes with airtight windows and doors, just turning on a dryer or kitchen exhaust fan can cause a dramatic reversal in the airflows of a house.

Airflows can be one factor affecting indoor air quality. I once compared 300 "sick" homes in which people were experiencing IAQ problems with 150 "control" homes I had inspected as part of real estate purchases. People suffering from asthma or allergies were almost twice as likely to be living in houses with hot-air heat, central air conditioning, or basement carpets. If you live in a home with any of these elements, you may want to read this book with particular care.

We now know that smoking is dangerous to health and that secondhand smoke irritates most people with asthma. We also know that off-gassing (the release of chemicals) from new rugs and new furniture can bother some people, and cockroach infestations can make allergy and asthma symptoms worse for others. In the chapters that follow, I deal with many IAQ issues, focusing primarily on sources of IAQ problems that are either microscopic or less well known.

Allergens are chemicals (often protein molecules) that may be associated with identifiable particles such as pollen, mold spores, bacteria, yeast, pet dander, and dust mite droppings and body parts. Many of the numerous particles suspended in the air can be identified only with sophisticated scientific equipment. To me, however, names are not the point. With my microscope I can identify many of the thousands of dust particles I collect, but I cannot identify them all. Even if I could, I would still need to take a vital step—figuring out the significance of these particles. If I collect samples in a space where people are suffering allergy or asthma symptoms, whatever I find is potentially relevant.

In the scientific method, a researcher forms a hypothesis and designs experiments to test it. If the hypothesis is that an IAQ problem exists only when the contaminants can be measured, are of a certain type, and reach a certain level, then the researcher goes about trying to prove or disprove the existence of the problem by measuring the concentration of a finite number of known pollutants. If this hypothesis is not supported by the sampling (and it usually isn't), then it is assumed that there is no IAQ problem, regardless of what people who spend time in the building are reporting (at this point sufferers may be advised to see a psychiatrist).

I approach indoor air quality from another angle. When people report asthma or allergy symptoms in an interior space, I assume there is a source for them. My task is to follow the clues that sampling provides and find the source. Usually I find it is the presence of *bioaerosols,* any suspended particulate in the air that comes from a living organism. For nonbioaerosol particulates, such as asbestos, which is an inorganic material, exposure would not result in immediate symptoms, and other types of testing are needed. Other toxic inorganic exposures that do not cause immediate symptoms nonetheless represent health risks. Testing for these substances may have to be done by a state or otherwise certified technician.

How do you know if you have allergies or asthma? There are some common symptoms, but often the picture is not clear and the presentation is not typical. Allergies are generally episodic, affecting the skin and the eyes, nose, and sinuses. Allergy in the skin often produces redness and itching and sometimes hives. Allergy in the nose, sinuses, and eyes (hay fever) often causes a runny nose, congestion, and burning and itching eyes. Asthma typically causes episodic respiratory symptoms, including wheezing and shortness of breath. Coughing is also a frequent symptom of asthma. People with asthma may notice that symptoms are triggered by specific allergens, like cats, or at particular times of the year. If you think you have an allergy or asthma, consult your physician. A generalist such as a family doctor may be able to make the diagnosis and start treatment or may refer you to a specialist.

This book is designed to help asthma and allergy sufferers as well as to serve as a preventive guide for all of us. I include information about spaces both inside and outside the home and explain why air quality problems might occur, make practical suggestions for eliminating them, and include stories about my many experiences helping people solve their IAQ problems. In the first two chapters, which set the scene, I include photomicrographs (photographs taken through a high-powered microscope) of some of the microscopic conditions and materials that can lead to IAQ problems. At the end of the book there is a glossary of technical vocabulary and scientific principles and a resource guide that will help you find IAQ information, products, and services.

Although I make comments about fungi and insects, I am neither a mycologist nor an entomologist. My comments are based largely on my observations. I apologize for any academic transgressions (for example, I use the genus and common name of organisms when I don't know the species).

I am not also a doctor and will not be giving medical advice; I would never tell people to disregard medical advice in favor of environmental measures. However, my experiences have led me to a firm belief that by better controlling the environments where we live and work, we can minimize the symptoms we or those we love may be suffering because of IAQ problems.

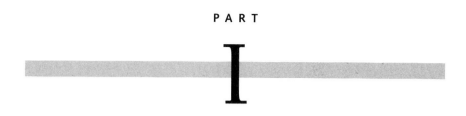

Setting the Scene

1

Cast of Characters

Let me begin by introducing the cast of characters, both visible and microscopic, that live in the world beneath our feet and under our noses. Members of the cast—organisms such as dust mites, mold, and yeast—and the creatures that feed on them can cause coughing, itchy eyes, and breathing difficulties. That's why controlling the growth of such organisms is often the key to eliminating indoor allergy symptoms and air quality problems.

DUST

House dust is its own universe, providing nutrition and shelter for an entire community of microscopic life. I can gather a lot of information about how someone lives by looking at the content of house dust. In my experience house dust consists mostly of human skin scales. The other particles present in dust depend on the inhabitants. If you have a bird, dog, or cat, for example, pet dander (skin scales) joins the mix. If you own a down quilt or down pillows, I'll find feather fibers from the bedding. I always find clothing fibers, and if a house has carpets I find carpet fibers. In or near a bathroom, either talc or cornstarch granules may be present in the air, depending on the type of body powder used. In a den where people munch snacks while watching TV, I find microscopic crumbs from cookies and potato chips in the dust from the sofa cushions. I find more soil particles and plant debris in the rooms where people first enter from the outside. If I'm sampling in the spring, I sometimes find pollen particles and other plant materials scattered throughout the house, but mostly in carpeting under the windows. If I find pollen in a carpet in the winter, I suspect the residents don't vacuum adequately.

Small particulates of dust, measuring approximately 0.00004 inch (under 1 micron), tend to remain suspended in still air for hours. Larger spherical particulates, above 0.002 inch (50 microns) in diameter, generally settle out of still air within seconds and form layers of visible dust on carpets, tables, shelves, and other surfaces. Thin, flat particulates (like skin scales) have more air resistance and stay aloft longer. Regardless of the shape of settled particulates, when we walk on carpets or move any stationary object, the settled dust particles are agitated and become airborne again.

If you want to see some of the particulates suspended in air, look closely at a beam of sunlight in a dimly lit room, or shine a flashlight at night. Of course to see what these particulates really are, you need more than a flashlight. I own two kinds of sampling instruments that help me collect particulates: an Allergenco air sampler and a Burkard sampler. An Allergenco sampler has a blower that pulls air through a narrow slit at a precise rate. After passing through the slit, the air stream hits a flat glass slide and is forced to take a sharp turn. The particulates in the air have so much momentum that they cannot make the turn with the air. They continue to travel in a straight path until they hit the slide and stick on its thin layer of grease. The instrument can be programmed to take multiple samples on a single slide, so I can compare them to see how the numbers and types of particulates change over time. I add biological stain to the particles, put a cover glass on the slide, and look at it with a microscope. With an Allergenco sampler, I can "see" the rise and fall in the concentration of aerosols (airborne particles) in the room air as the level of activity changes. A Burkard sampler is a similar device that also collects dust particles on a greased microscope slide, but it can take only one sample at a time on each slide.

In a clean home with hardwood floors and leather furniture, I do not see a high level of dust in my samples, even with a reasonable amount of room activity. In a home with wall-to-wall carpeting and stuffed furniture, my air samples are sometimes so thickly layered with dust that it's difficult to distinguish the different particulates. If you are in a room with a hundred people, the air will contain shed skin scales and pet dander, among other suspended particulates. Each person will inhale these particulates with every breath. For-

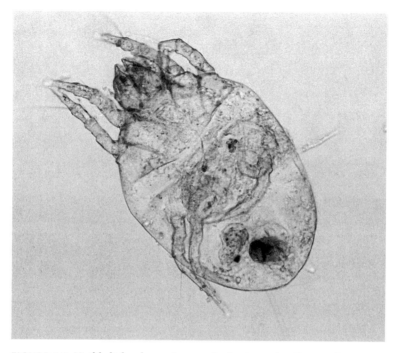

FIGURE 1.1. Visible light photomicrograph of a dust mite. Even with a microscope, live mites are very difficult to find in dust, because they are small, translucent, and very shy. This mite came from a sample of vacuumed carpet dust and tried to escape from a silverfish that was devouring the mite's kin. The dark round spot at its abdomen is probably a fecal pellet. Photomicrographs of dust mites taken with a scanning electron microscope (as in Figure 1.2) make them look formidable. In fact, they are delicate, consisting of a fragile bag of liquid with four legs on each side, a mouth at one end, and an anus at the other. (200× light)

tunately most such particulates are benign, and the human respiratory system (including the nose, trachea, and lungs) is designed to capture them and then remove or destroy them.

DUST MITES

Dust is home to dust mites, considered one of the most common causes of allergy and asthma symptoms in the world. Dust mites are about 0.01 inch (0.25 millimeter) long and are usually invisible to the naked eye, though you could see a mite crawling on a black background. When I sample in houses infested

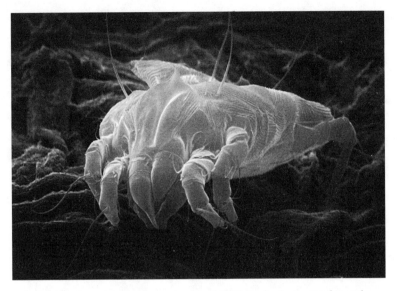

FIGURE 1.2. Scanning electron micrograph (SEM) of a dust mite skin. Like most insects, dust mites hatch from eggs. The nymph that crawls out molts several times before achieving its final adult form. The dust mite shown here is actually a cast-off skin from a molt. (650× SEM)

with dust mites, I am likely to find microscopic mite legs and other body parts, as well as mite fecal pellets, in the air after surfaces have been disturbed. (There will be many references in the book to insect fecal material, sometimes called *frass*; frass is one of the major allergenic components in dust.)

It takes about a month for a dust mite egg to hatch and the mite to mature to an adult. An adult female mite may live another month and produce two hundred eggs. Mites lay their eggs in skin-laden house dust; we shed about an ounce (approximately 30 grams) of skin scales each month, so the food for mites is in essentially infinite supply. Our sloughed-off skin scales are small enough to slip through the cotton weave of pillowcases, sheets, and mattress pads, and they gather inside our pillows and mattresses. You could beat a bed pillow for half an hour and there would still be enough food left for thousands of mites. Even our clothing can harbor mites and thus be a source of contamination. A Canadian study found that a heavy winter coat that is frequently worn but rarely washed can acquire a significant population of mites, several per square inch. Items like these can cause allergy symptoms for the wearer, another sensitized family member, or even a coworker who breathes the particulates that become airborne as the item is moved. When we store such clothing in bureaus or closets, the mites and their allergens may be dispersed into the environment.

Dust mites need moisture to flourish. In bed we provide this moisture from our skin and our breath. When we breathe into our pillows, mites (if present) congregate to imbibe the moisture. Warm quilts or thick, soft mattress pads soak up our body moisture and thus are often teeming with microscopic life. Those of us who sweat a great deal or sleep under piles of blankets or in overheated bedrooms risk greater infestations. Conversely, people who use only a light covering or do not sweat much are less likely to have mites in their mattresses. Dust mites colonize thicker materials, where moisture levels tend to remain more constant. Thinner materials dry out faster and thus do not provide the best living and breeding conditions for mites.

The Variety of Mites

Dust mites such as *Dermatophagoides pteronyssinus* and *Dermatophagoides farinae* are only two of over a dozen common species of mites found in houses. One mite, *Cheyletus eruditus*, preys on dust mites. Another, *Glycyphagus domesticus*, is called grocer's itch mite because it thrives on flour and wheat.

Tyroglyphus farinae—called a storage mite—also lives in stored grains. I read about two cases of allergy to storage mites. In one case a child had a severe asthmatic reaction in a pizzeria after the raw dough coated with dry flour was flattened and flung spinning into the air. When the flour became airborne, mite allergens were dispersed. In the second case a child ate food made from contaminated flour. I know someone with a severe mite allergy who occasionally falls into a stupor and sleeps for several hours after eating a sandwich. Although there is no apparent pattern to these incidents, I suspect they occur when mite-contaminated flour is used.

In one type of test for allergies, small amounts of carefully prepared extracts of potential allergens are introduced under the skin with a needle prick. If the skin reacts, the person is said to have a positive reaction to that allergen. A negative reaction to one type of dust mite does not rule out allergy to other species, and unfortunately allergy testing is not available for many common species of mites. Mites' fecal pellets, whatever the species, are the major source of allergens, because they may contain allergenic materials such as mite digestive enzymes or mold spores.

The Climate for Mites

Moisture is visible as liquid water but invisible as water vapor in air. *Relative humidity* is a measure of how much water vapor is in the air compared with the maximum amount of moisture the air can contain at a given temperature—how close air is to being saturated. Air at 80 percent relative humidity can still contain more moisture. Air at 100 percent relative humidity looks just the same but can hold no more water vapor. Relative humidity is an important concept to understand in the battle against indoor air quality problems, because microscopic life flourishes at higher relative humidity.

In relative humidity above 70 percent, for example, mites can grow in dust without added moisture from our bodies (at lower relative humidity, mites congregate in clusters to conserve their moisture). As the relative humidity rises, dust mites increase their rate of reproduction, intake of skin scales, and defecation. This is significant because, as I noted above, dust mite fecal pellets are the major source of mite allergens. In a mite-infested environment, over 100,000 mite fecal pellets may be found in a gram of dust, and these pellets can become airborne and be inhaled.

When relative humidity is 100 percent, water vapor will condense onto any surface that is below the temperature of the air around it. For example, imagine you are sitting outside in Florida on a 75°F day, and the relative humidity of the air around you is 100 percent. If you are holding a drink at 76°F, moisture will not condense on the glass. If you lower the temperature of the liquid below 75°F with an ice cube, you see condensation on the glass.

The temperature of air that is at 100 percent relative humidity is called the *dew point*. Why is this relevant to IAQ concerns? As you will see in later chapters, by keeping the relative humidity in our homes as low as we can, we keep the dew point low and thus reduce the chances of air quality problems due to dust mites, mold, and other organisms.

FROM MITES TO MOLD

Mold needs the same conditions for growth as mites: moisture and nutrients. Some mites (for example, *Tyrophagus putrescentiae*) are often found foraging

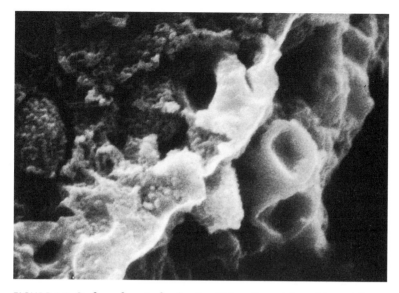

FIGURE 1.3. Surface of a mite fecal pellet. This pellet was found in a sticky tape sample taken from the back of a basement door covered with *Aspergillus* mold. Numerous mite body parts were also found. At the left are two *Aspergillus* spores embedded within the pellet. The homeowner's fiancé experienced allergy problems every time he opened the door to the basement. (7,000× SEM)

on mold growth. In basements where the relative humidity is over 70 percent, the foundation walls and floors are often blackened by mold colonies that are home to mold-eating mites. In one basement room, an entire wall was covered by what appeared to be only mold. When I looked at a sample of the dark dust, however, I found that it consisted of mold spores, nearly all of them clumped within mite fecal pellets! The fecal pellets of mites that eat mold contain mold spores or bits of chewed mold. If the fecal pellets get wet, viable mold spores within may germinate.

Molds are *fungi* (sing. *fungus*). Mushrooms too are fungi. The microscopic plantlike "chefs" that help convert grapes to wine and wort to beer are also fungi. One genus of mold, *Penicillium*, comprises hundreds of known species: some produce the antibiotic penicillin, and others turn milk curd into cheese. Some species of *Penicillium* create the blue-green growth found on long-forgotten oranges at the back of a refrigerator drawer.

Most fungi reproduce by creating spores, microscopic cells that these or-

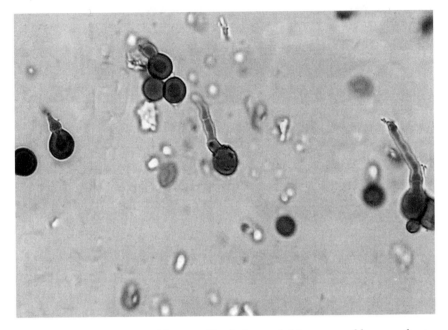

FIGURE 1.4. Germinating mold spores. The dark round objects are mold spores, three of which are germinating. When moisture conditions are appropriate, a spore germinates by sending out a hyphal foot. The spore at the left has just started to germinate while the other two with longer hyphae started growing sooner. These spores are from mold growing on the lower part of a bedroom wall, hidden behind the headboard of the bed. (1,000× light)

ganisms generate in great numbers. Some spores grow in clumps that are stuck together. Others grow in long, fragile chains that are easily dispersed into the air if the fungus is disturbed. If adequate moisture is present when a spore lands on a suitable food source, it uses nutrients stored within it to start growing. The spore sends out a small extension called a *hypha* (pl. *hyphae*), similar to the root from a germinating seed. This is the beginning of a mold colony.

Unlike an animal, which digests food within itself, fungi secrete enzymes from the growing tips of the hyphae to digest food sources outside the organism. The resulting nutrients diffuse into the organism through the cell wall at the tip. As the hypha elongates, it splits and lengthens, eventually creating a complex network of hyphae called a *mycelium*. Often the mycelium is white and furry, but as many fungal colonies mature they may acquire the color of their spores—black, yellow, brown, or green. Within days a single spore can easily produce a mature colony containing millions of spores.

Mold can't use inorganic materials such as concrete or rock for food, but it can consume anything organic, or carbon based, that lands on these surfaces. Mold can grow on dust, fruit, paper, cotton, soap, oil, paint, and wood. In buildings, many of the materials mold grows on (such as wood framing, wallpaper, fabrics, drywall, and cardboard boxes) contain *cellulose,* a plant substance. Cellulose is a *polymer* (a long-chain molecule) of glucose. The starch we eat is also a polymer of glucose. Our digestive enzymes break starch down into individual glucose molecules that taste sweet. This process starts in the mouth, so a cracker develops a sweet taste as we chew it.

Humans can't digest cellulose, because the glucose molecules are linked or bonded differently than they are in starch, but fungi can. Wood is primarily a composite of cellulose and *lignin,* another complex plant substance that even some fungi cannot digest. Wood consists of a network of tubes like a bundle

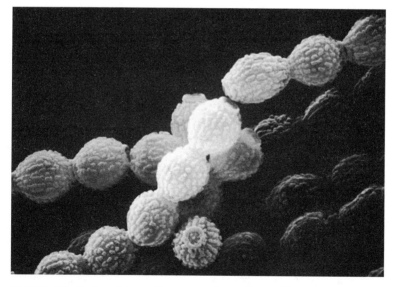

FIGURE 1.5. Chains of *Aspergillus* spores. *Aspergillus* mold spores are produced in a long, fragile chain that resembles a pop-bead necklace. With very slight physical disturbances, the spores separate and become airborne. (5,000× SEM)

of drinking straws. When a mold spore lands on damp wood, it's like a fly landing on a lollipop. Sugar! The hyphae elongate and grow through the hollow tubes of the wood structure, breaking down the cellulose, metabolizing the sugar, and destroying the strawlike walls, or "rotting" the wood. When the wood dries out, the mold stops growing and may even die. What is left behind consists of, among other things, mold growth (including spores and hyphae), partially digested cellulose, and the undigested lignin. When the wood gets wet the mold may start to grow again.

People who are sensitized to spores will react allergically if they breathe in airborne mold spores. They may cough, sneeze, experience eye irritation, or wheeze. But mold can bother people who do not have mold allergy at all. The content of every mold spore is different, but the cell walls are similar. It is now believed that components of the cell wall, called *glucans,* of all mold spores can inflame lung tissue.

Mycotoxins

Mycotoxins are the chemicals fungi make as they grow and process nutrients (*myco* means fungus). Scientists do not yet know what functions mycotoxins may serve, but the more closely investigators look at different species of molds, the more often they find mycotoxins. Though most traditional mycotoxin poisoning (*mycotoxicosis*) is associated with eating toxic mushrooms or mold-contaminated grains, it now seems likely that inhaling spores containing mycotoxins can also be hazardous.

Aspergillus flavus, a common mold that grows on nuts and grains and can be found in homes, can produce aflatoxin B_1 (a kind of mycotoxin), one of several chemicals that are among the most carcinogenic compounds known. The black mold *Stachybotrys chartarum,* commonly found on chronically damp drywall, can also produce a series of mycotoxins (called tricothecenes) that are very poisonous. In the 1930s Russian horses started dying in large numbers. Symptoms included inflammation of the skin and respiratory tract and hemorrhaging. Death sometimes occurred within twenty-four hours of the time symptoms appeared. The horses' feed was found to be contaminated with *Stachybotrys chartarum.* In the mid-1990s, based on evidence from cases at Cleveland's Rainbow Babies and Children's Hospital, Dr. Dorr Dearborn associated *Stachybotrys* with *pulmonary hemosiderosis* (bleeding in the lungs).

Though some disputed his conclusions, Dr. Dearborn concluded that several infant deaths were caused by this mold. In the same decade, a house in Texas became so contaminated by *Stachybotrys* that the family had to abandon the property and bulldoze the house. The husband experienced memory loss, and the child became asthmatic. The man who was investigating the case threw up for hours after spending thirty minutes in the contaminated building.

Mildew

Familiar forms of fungi include the mildew often seen in bathrooms and on basement walls. Mildew can grow on nutrients in soap film, paper, and paint or in dust on a surface. If you find mildew growing anywhere in your home, don't ignore it, because it too produces spores that can become airborne.

One family asked me to help them determine the source of a strong mildew odor in their home. The odor originated in the old basement carpet, and they removed it. The smell went away, and they installed new nylon carpeting, which was supposed to be nonallergenic. Two months later they went on a

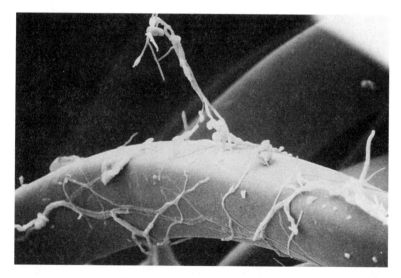

FIGURE 1.6. A carpet fiber with mold. This fiber from a nylon carpet had mold hyphae creeping like vine along the surface. Most of the hyphae are wrapped around the thicker carpet fiber, but one portion projects upward. Other hyphae not visible in the photo had spread from one nylon fiber to the next. The invisible mold growth gave the nearly new carpet its musty odor. (450× SEM)

two-week summer vacation, leaving the central air conditioning on. When they returned, they again noticed a mildew odor. I went once more to look at the house and found that the condensate pump on the air conditioner had broken, allowing water to leak out of the basement mechanical closet and into the new carpeting.

Curious as to what had occurred, I cut out a small piece of the carpet and took it to a scanning electron microscopist. I had expected to find mold growing at the bottom of the fibers in the backing, where the dust ultimately accumulates. The microscopist and I spent an hour examining the fingernail-sized sample, and much to our surprise we found mold at the top of the nylon fiber loops rather than at the bottom. Since the carpet was new, the dust that had settled from the air onto the nylon fibers had not yet fallen down to the backing, and the germinating spores had sent out hyphae where the food source was. The microscopist and I could see the hyphae growing like ivy on a telephone pole, clinging to carpet fibers and lengthening as they grew toward successive dust particulates and consumed them. That the carpeting material was nylon (and sold as nonallergenic) did not deter mold growth within it, for as is often the case with synthetic carpeting, the mold was consuming the dust rather than the carpet fibers. The family eliminated the problem by replacing the condensate pump and the contaminated section of carpet near the mechanical closet.

CARPET CRITTERS

It was not until the 1960s that the medical community had sufficient evidence to accept the theory that dust mites cause allergy. Now physicians recognize that fecal material and body parts from other insects may also cause allergy and asthma symptoms: cockroaches are a well-known example. In addition to mold growth and dust mites, I have found silverfish, booklice, and carpet beetles (dermestids) in some of my clients' carpeting. Except for entomologists and pest control operators, few people have ever seen or heard of a carpet beetle, yet these very common pests may cause symptoms as well.

Carpet Beetles

There are a variety of household beetle pests, but two common ones are the black carpet beetle (*Attagenus megatoma*) and the varied carpet beetle

(*Athrenus verbasci*). The adults of both species are about 0.12 inch (3 millimeters) long, but the former is black and the latter is multicolored (white, yellowish, and brownish scales). Carpet beetles lay their eggs in larger dead animals and insects: a dead moth is a favorite place. The eggs hatch and produce young that *molt* (shed the outer layer) into hairy larvae that feed on anything that contains protein, including hair, fur, and animals. Like other larvae, they have voracious appetites and do nothing but eat, defecate, and molt. If you move a piece of furniture, you may find the carcass of a moth or bee on the floor surrounded by a circular thin layer of brown dust an inch (2.5 centimeters) or so in diameter. This dust could be the frass (fecal pellets) of a carpet beetle larva that has fed on the dead insect. Many valuable collections of butterflies and other insects have been turned to frass by these creatures.

Carpet beetle larvae love hair and are the scourge of museums with mounted specimens. They don't care where the hair comes from: it can be

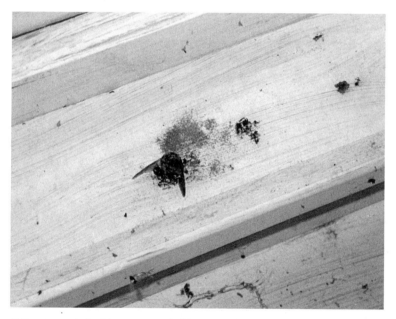

FIGURE 1.7. A dead bee surrounded by carpet beetle frass. An adult carpet beetle laid eggs in a bee that had died at an attic window. The larvae hatched and partially ate the body of the bee. The oval dust layer in front of the dead bee consists entirely of carpet beetle frass. Droppings in the frass contained chewed pieces of bee.

from a mighty stuffed lion, from the wool fibers in an Oriental rug, or from your body or the body of a beloved pet. In dust samples from carpeting and beds, I have seen hairs that larvae have gnawed to points resembling roughly sharpened pencils. In the fecal pellets of these creatures, you can see the chewed bits of whatever they have been feeding on.

Although these fecal pellets are far too large to become airborne, about 0.0055 inch (140 microns), I was curious to know if they could be broken apart. I crushed a pellet and accidentally breathed in the dust. My throat swelled and I immediately had trouble breathing. Since that experience, I read about research by a doctor from Spain who notes allergy to carpet beetles. In *Urban Entomology*, Walter Ebeling also describes cases of allergy to dermestids, possibly due to the beetles' hairs and body parts.

Carpet beetle frass may even be useful to crime investigators. I received an e-mail message from a forensic chemist who had been searching the Internet for information on carpet beetles when she found my home page. She won-

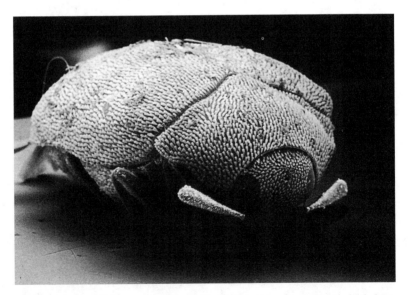

FIGURE 1.8. An adult carpet beetle. Apparently another carpet beetle had already found a dead moth before the moth was placed in a closed plastic box and had laid its eggs within the moth's body. Soon two hairy beetle larvae appeared and fed on the moth for weeks. After a few months, two mature carpet beetles emerged. (40× SEM)

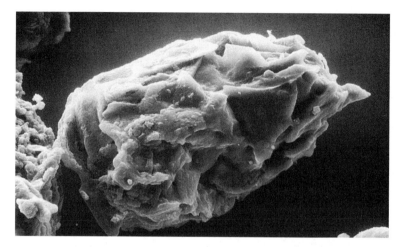

FIGURE 1.9. Carpet beetle fecal pellet with pieces of chewed-up bee. This is a fecal pellet from the carpet beetle frass, deposited around the dead bee shown in figure 1.7. The triangular shape near the right end of the pellet is probably a piece of the bee's exoskeleton. Other similar bits can be seen edge-on along the surface of the fecal pellet. The material in clumps at the pellet surface consists of crystals of nitrogen-containing waste. (600× SEM)

dered if it would be possible to determine whether the chewed-up hair in carpet beetle frass contained hair dye. She was very circumspect about why she needed this information, but I can only assume that the police were attempting to identify a decomposed body by looking at the hair fragments in the frass.

Moths

Wool carpeting and clothing can attract moths, and moth fecal material and body parts may cause allergic symptoms in some people. I had my own problem with wool moths. My brother and his wife gave us an imported woven wool wall hanging containing muted shades of red, gold, and brown that matched our decor. One day my wife noticed that one of the tassels had fallen off the bottom. She took a closer look at the fabric and noticed that all the tassels were frayed; in some spots the yarn had been reduced to the thickness of a thread. She looked at the back of the fabric, and to her horror she found hundreds of quivering moths and writhing larvae embedded in the material.

The hanging was directly above a radiator. I put on a fine-particle face mask, threw the hanging away, then vacuumed up and saved the dust on the

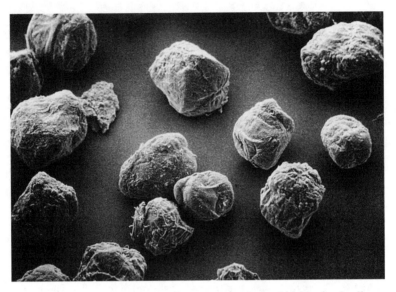

FIGURE 1.10. Wool moth fecal pellets. An individual pebblelike fecal pellet from a wool moth larva has the color of the ingested dyed fiber. People see brown dust, but under a microscope the different colors become visible. If you have a wool moth infestation, you could wipe up thousands of such pellets with a quick swipe of your hand or dust cloth. (50× SEM)

floor below and behind the radiator. With a light microscope, I could see that the dust consisted of nearly pure larval frass. The fecal pellets had different colors, the same muted tones as the hanging. At very high magnification (30,000 power) with an electron microscope I could see that the surface of each pellet consisted of nearly spherical crystals called *spherules* (possibly containing *guanine,* a chemical insects excrete), all bound together by some unknown coating. Later I tapped a box containing some of the frass and took a Burkard sample of the air above it. I found some of the approximately 0.00004 inch (1 micron) spherules in the air, and I surmised that my tapping had dislodged them from the surface of the fecal pellets. Although the intact pellets were too large to become airborne, the spherules were not, and these may have contained surface allergens.

"Litterature"

The dust that has settled on books seems to bother many people with allergies. There is nothing really special about the dust on books except that it often sits there longer than the dust on other surfaces. Once the book is disturbed, particulates become airborne.

We may think of the words inside as intellectual nourishment, but the particulates that settle on the outside of the book provide real sustenance for a wide variety of insect life. When I look at book dust, I may find booklice, settled pollen and mold spores, spider silk, mites or their body parts, and insect fecal material. In book dust that has nurtured insects, I find chewed pollen grains or fecal pellets consisting entirely of partially digested pollen.

Booklice, also called *psocids,* are about 0.06 inch (1.5 millimeters) long and are sometimes found feeding on books that are stored in damp basements. Psocids aren't really lice, but they resemble them. Some people believe psocids are attracted to the starch in the book bindings, for they also infest stored grains that contain starch. I met my first booklouse while I was reading at my desk and saw a small buff-colored bug scurrying across the page. I trapped the unknown creature on a piece of sticky tape and placed the tape on a glass slide to view under my microscope. While I was observing the insect, it ejected a

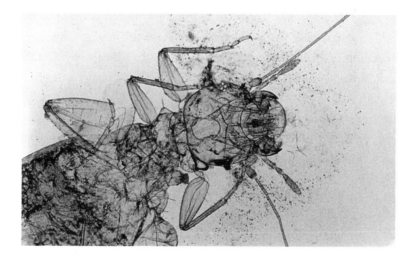

FIGURE 1.11. A booklouse. In a year-long study in Madrid, sticky traps placed in bathrooms, kitchens, and inside windows captured hundreds of booklice. One study in Germany found that approximately one-third of city dwellers tested were allergic to booklice. (100× light)

small dark pellet, about 0.003 inch (76 microns) in diameter, from the end of its abdomen.

Suddenly I had the unique opportunity to observe an uncontaminated fecal pellet from a known source. I managed to get the pellet to adhere to a tiny drop of water, suspended at the end of a pin, and to transfer the drop to a microscope slide. I crushed the pellet, added acid fuchsin stain, and observed that it contained skin scales and mold spores. I thus discovered that these insects, in addition to eating bookbindings, forage in the dust for mold spores and our skin scales, as mites do.

Unlike mite fecal pellets, which are known allergens, the entire booklouse fecal pellet is too large to become readily airborne. However, I did see respirable crystals (possibly coated with allergens) drifting away from the surface of the pellet before I crushed it. This is all still new territory for allergy research, but there have been recent reports in the medical literature of allergy to booklice.

BIGGER PESTS
Spiders

Although some people regard spiders in their homes as beneficial, most know how poisonous a black widow or brown recluse can be. Some have severe reactions to the bites of less threatening spiders. I also believe spiders are a source of fecal allergens. If you look under a spiderweb, you will find clusters of white dots resembling paint spatters about 0.04 to 0.08 inch (1 to 2 millimeters) in diameter, some containing a dark bull's-eye. These clusters are the spider's fecal material. The dots consist of microscopic (about 0.00004 inch or 1 micron) crystals that can become airborne if disturbed by our footsteps. I think that though the crystals consist of almost pure guanine, each is stuck to its neighbors by an allergenic coating, possibly containing spider proteins.

To obtain spider droppings for a scanning electron micrograph, I set up a blind in the corner of my office where I had noticed a small web with a spider in the middle. I placed a petri dish directly beneath the spider. It must have seen its own reflection in the shiny surface, because it jumped down and attacked the petri dish. I was thrilled that I had an aggressive subject, since the spider would be energetic in capturing prey and would thus yield my much sought after fecal material. I even placed a small nightlight on the floor near the web to lure prey to the spot. Unfortunately, before I could gather any results my wife swooped away the entire apparatus to make way for her vacuuming.

I repeated the experiment in the winter, but this time I hid the petri dish in a closet and left it beneath a spiderweb for a month. When I collected the dish at last, I found it contained not only spider droppings but also four dried-up booklice the spider had preyed on. This experiment provided not only fecal material but insight into house ecology, since I was reminded of the unseen battles that take place in the hidden corners of our homes every day. The experiment also reinforced my belief that spider droppings may be allergenic, because as soon as the electron microscopist disturbed the material I started to cough and wheeze.

The presence of many spiders in your home means too much moisture. All living things consist mostly of water. If an insect dries out, it dies. Many small insects don't drink water, so they have to extract it from their food or absorb it from the air through the exterior layers of their bodies. Spiders get their liquids from what they eat, and mites are on their menu. In turn, mites (as well as booklice and many other small household pests) absorb moisture directly from the humidity in the air. So much for the theory that spiders are a healthy sign.

Cockroaches

Cockroaches, particularly prevalent in cities, are one of the pests recognized as causing asthma symptoms. I recall reading a case study about a woman with asthma who was severely allergic to cockroaches. Her apartment was infested, and she was hospitalized with symptoms. She was warned not to go home before the roaches were eliminated. Unfortunately she couldn't afford to have the apartment properly treated and cleaned. When she moved back in, she became acutely ill and died.

Once while I was living in a dormitory, I walked over to a large paper train schedule taped to the wall near our common kitchen. As I pointed to the departure time, I touched the paper. A cockroach dropped to the floor and scurried off. Horrified but curious, I lifted the edge of the schedule and peeked behind it. I had accidentally discovered a roach *harborage* or shelter, where there were hundreds of motionless insects, packed nearly pest to pest. Cockroaches spend the daylight hours in their harborage, attracted to each other and to the location by aggregation pheromones in the abundant feces they leave there.

A cockroach harborage is usually near a supply of food and moisture, most commonly in kitchens and bathrooms. Cockroaches prefer narrow spaces where both the tops and bottoms of their bodies can be in contact with porous surfaces such as wood. They are often found in the dead space between a kitchen cabinet and the wall or in crevices associated with shelves holding food. Harborages commonly are under appliances such as stoves or refrigerators or in appliance insulation. In larger infestations the insects can be found even in televisions and dressers. Cockroaches tend to move about at the floor/wall joint rather than in the middle of rooms, so the best way to determine the extent of an infestation is to set out sticky traps along likely travel routes. By doing this methodically, you can even find the harborage.

Cockroaches are nocturnal and forage at night. They will eat just about anything, including garbage. The best way to minimize the likelihood of cockroach infestations is to store all foods in closed containers (don't leave pet food out overnight). Cockroach allergens may be found in food where roaches have foraged; if you eat the food, you ingest the allergens. When kitchen or pantry dust containing cockroach droppings and body parts is disturbed, these allergens can become airborne and be inhaled (though scientists have found that much of roach allergen aerosol is on particles larger than 0.0004 inch [10 microns], so these allergens remain airborne only briefly). It is also believed that cockroaches can spread certain illnesses. For example, if the cockroaches eat food contaminated with *Salmonella,* the bacteria that cause food poisoning, viable *Salmonella* can be found in the roach feces. Should this fecal material end up in food eaten by humans, the roach may transmit food poisoning.

An adult of one of the more common species of cockroaches, *Blattella germanica* or the German cockroach, grows to about 0.5 inch (12.7 millimeters). These creatures are quite hardy and can live up to twenty days without food or water. This means roaches can move into your home on furniture that has been purchased from a yard sale or stored in a moving truck. After German cockroaches mate, the female produces an egg case containing about thirty eggs. She carries the case, which resembles a brown purse about 0.3 by 0.1 inch (8 by 3 millimeters), until the eggs are ready to hatch (in about a month).

The *nymphs* that hatch are still immature, about 0.12 inch (3 millimeters) long, and look gray to black. Over about sixty days, they will molt six or seven times before becoming adults. An individual roach may live two hundred days, and a single female can produce up to three hundred offspring. Within a year, under warm and moist conditions, a few roaches can theoretically grow into a colony of millions.

One of my clients told me that friends of his with a significant cockroach infestation discovered, in the middle of the winter, that the roaches were nesting in the gasket of their dishwasher. They decided the simplest way to kill the pests was to freeze them. They disconnected the dishwasher and put it outside, and this eliminated the problem in the appliance. They continued to have roaches in the kitchen, however, so they applied their special treatment to the entire house. They drained the plumbing, turned off the heat, and left the house vacant. By freezing the pests, they were able to get rid of their roaches without using pesticides. If you live in a warm climate, however, shipping your home to Alaska is probably not an option. A borate-based pesticide (based on boric acid) would be a relatively safe choice, since these pesticides contain no solvents and do not evaporate.

Ants

I have never heard that people have allergic reactions to ants unless bitten. If you do have an ant infestation, I don't recommend liquid or spray pesticides, because chronic exposure to them can make humans chemically sensitive, particularly if they are incorrectly applied. If you must use pesticide, choose ant baits or a borate pesticide. Sticky paper traps can give you an idea of the kinds of insects that are in the kitchen (if you really want to know).

We once had a red ant problem in our kitchen that I discovered when I opened a cabinet that rested on the floor. I was reaching for the cereal box when I noticed that the walls, shelves, and packages were crawling with small red ants. There was a gap between two floorboards that ran under the cabinet. Inside the crack, the ants were moving in two well-organized lines: one in, one out. Ants in the "out" line were carrying bits of my breakfast away to the nest. They disappeared under the baseboard at the outside wall. When I went into the basement the marching battalions reappeared, traveling in opposite directions in the same two lines horizontally along the sill toward the framing beneath the kitchen door. Directly beneath the threshold, the line turned upward. When I went upstairs and outside the kitchen, I could see the army crawling up and down the trim board under the threshold and along a joist beneath the exterior deck. At the end of the joists, they marched along a vertical deck support post that went into the soil. The ants were exiting and entering from the bottom of a piece of flagstone resting on the soil next to the post. I lifted the flagstone, and there were my cornflakes.

Often the best solution is patience. Follow the ants as they carry the food home, then destroy the nest.

Carpenter Ants

Sometimes air quality problems are caused not by the pests themselves but by the damp conditions that attract them. When you see evidence of insect infestation, you may also find moist wood or another environment that is not only attractive to pests but also conducive to the growth of mold or other allergens. Carpenter ants are one pest that can signal excessive moisture.

Carpenter ants carve out their nests in wet wood because, like most insects, they thrive in humid environments. During one of my first home inspections, I saw dozens of carpenter ants crawling down a water pipe that ran through a hole under the kitchen sink. There was a leak in the pipe, and the wood beneath was rotting. I could see this was no surprise to the owners; instead of fixing the leak, they had covered a filing cabinet in the basement with plastic. Each black ant was about an inch long and had wings. These were the reproductive queens, produced by an ant colony in the spring. Each queen was capable of starting a new carpenter ant nest. Fixing the leak would have kept the filing cabinet dry and the carpenter ant nest in the yard where it belonged.

Another homeowner called me because she was plagued by big black carpenter ants in her kitchen. She joked that when she baked cookies for her children she had to set aside extra ones as decoys for the ants. The ants moved in soon after completion of their kitchen addition, an octagonal space containing built-in benches around a table. The roof had a very low slope, the gutters were narrow, and there was no overhang. When water overflowed the gutters, it thus ran directly down the siding rather than away from it. I lifted the hinged seat in the new kitchen addition and measured the moisture content of the drywall with a Tramex meter; the reading suggested excessive moisture. The most likely source was rain running down the outside wall.

I recommended they remove some of the drywall from inside the seats to see if there was decay. I later received a hysterical phone call. At the bottom of each stud bay they opened was a seething, checkered mass of black ants and white ant eggs. Their contractor removed the bottom few inches of drywall from all sides of the addition, and in each bay he found a carpenter ant nest. Fortunately, though the scene was hideous there was no damage to the wood. The ants had not needed to chew their way into or through the wood, because there were plenty of small gaps and spaces for them to enter the stud bays, and the bays themselves were roomy enough for the nests. The fiberglass insulation kept the temperature constant, and the leaks kept the humidity at Floridian levels.

Another woman I spoke with unfortunately took a different approach to a carpenter ant invasion in her kitchen, though one that many people undertake without ill effects. She decided to drill holes and spray volatile pesticide (a liquid that evaporates) into every stud bay in the kitchen. She is now chemically sensitive and cannot tolerate even perfume. The woman is convinced that her sensitivity began shortly after her overexposure to the pesticide.

BACK TO THE INVISIBLE
Bacteria and Yeast

So far we've discussed relatively well known sources of allergens such as mites, mold, and cockroaches. Bacteria, which we know cause respiratory and other infections, can also lead to allergy-type reactions. *Actinomycetes*, organisms that produce small spores and grow like mold, are actually filamentous bacteria. Actinomycetes are present in soil and produce its characteristic earthy odor. Chronic inhalation of actinomycete spores can lead to the pulmonary disease "farmer's lung," a type of hypersensitivity pneumonitis. The yeast we add to dough to lighten bread is another microorganism. Some types of yeast cause allergy.

Mate Allergy or Self-Allergy?

I've always been intrigued by the idea of becoming allergic to your mate. More than once I've heard people say their allergies started after their partners moved in. Recent papers in the medical literature point to a possible scientific reason: several common fungi called *dermatophytes* can cause medical conditions such as dermatitis and dandruff.

These fungi can exist in two forms. In a petri dish culture they grow like other molds; but on human skin they revert to a yeast form. Instead of growing in colonies and producing hyphae, individual yeast cells simply divide by budding into parent and daughter cells. These yeast cells are the size of mold spores and thus can be breathed in. Fortunately dermatophytes, unlike mold spores, do not easily become airborne, because they adhere to the oily surface of the skin scales they grow on. Recently two proteins that are allergens have been identified on the surface of yeast cells. One study found that almost 10 percent of hairdressers in Finland react with allergic symptoms to the yeasts that cause dandruff and dermatitis.

I learned about inhalant yeast allergy when a client asked me to investigate his apartment, where he had been experiencing severe asthma symptoms. He was desperate, because after he spent time at home his breathing became so labored that he could barely walk to his car or go out to shop for food. Whenever he was away for more than two days, he felt better.

I was pretty sure I would find mold and mites, but I was surprised. The man was a fastidious housekeeper; there was little dust anywhere, and I could find no source of excess moisture. Yet the dust samples I collected from his bedding and favorite TV chair were full of skin scales covered with yeast. Walking on the carpet also produced large numbers of individual respirable yeast cells. Although I had no trouble breathing in the apartment, he was convinced his home was contaminated. I can only assume that the yeast was subsisting on the skin scales shed by the man's body. In this case the man may well have been allergic to something that his own body was "feeding."

The bad news is that it is difficult to test for this particular yeast allergy, because the allergens are not very stable and thus can't be easily stored in solution and kept in the doctor's refrigerator for study. The good news is that their instability makes them easier to destroy. I suspect that thoroughly treating all the furniture and carpeting with dry steam would destroy most of the unstable allergens (see "Dry" Steam in chapter 14). Dry steam is water vapor alone, without liquid water. At the temperature of steam, many allergens are "cooked."

BOOKS

- Books should be vacuumed periodically with a HEPA vacuum (a high-efficiency particulate arrestance vacuum cleaner, described in chapter 14).
- If you are particularly sensitive, consider storing your books in closed cases.
- Be careful about accepting or buying books that may have been stored in damp, closed spaces. Even if you find that rare book you've been searching for, if it smells moldy, don't bring it home.

PESTS

- Used furniture or furniture that has been stored in infested spaces may contain cockroaches; be wary about introducing such furniture into your home.
- Avoid volatile pesticides. Have wooden structural components in basements treated with borate preservative to minimize mold and insect infestations.

The Stage, Set, and Crew

In the first chapter I introduced a cast of characters, both microscopic and visible. Now think about the stage on which these creatures act out their roles: our rugs, furniture, and bedding; our pets, our plants, and even our own bodies. Whether the drama that unfolds is a tragedy or a comedy depends on conditions *we* help create.

CARPETING

Many carpets and rugs are fine, but some are fiber jungles alive with mites, carpet beetles, and mold, all peppered with pet dander. Even new carpeting and rugs can be contaminated if they have been stored in damp or dirty spaces. If your rug or carpeting is used, you may not know whether the previous owner or tenant had a dog or cat or whether the carpeting is infested with mold or mites.

On numerous occasions I have taken samples of the air above Oriental rugs after patting them to disturb the dust. One woman had trouble breathing in the office corner of her living room. The dust from the rug contained a significant growth of *Aspergillus* mold. She had bought the rug from an antiques dealer and had no idea who had owned it or under what conditions the rug had been stored. In a family with allergies or asthma, previously owned rugs must be chosen with great care and professionally cleaned before use.

Both rugs and wall-to-wall carpets can harbor the same ecosystems, but there are two significant differences. A contaminated rug can be rolled up (carefully!), removed, and professionally washed. Carpets, on the other hand, are usually left in place far too long. If vacuumed infrequently or washed by amateurs (see chapter 14 on cleaning carpets), carpeting can become contaminated. Just as pillows and mattresses emit allergens when compressed, carpet fibers can emit thousands of airborne irritants with every step. And once present in carpet dust, some allergens and mycotoxins can cause symptoms for the life of the carpet.

Moisture and carpets do not make a good combination. I received a call from a management company that was dealing with a complaint from a first-floor tenant. The building was slab on grade, meaning there was no basement, and the floor of the unit was concrete. Though the management company had replaced all the carpeting in the bedroom before the tenant moved in two months earlier, he claimed mold grew on his shoes when he kept them under his bed. I was very skeptical. I took room air samples and bulk samples of the dust under the bed for microscopic analysis. There were spores in the air, which didn't surprise me, but I was amazed to see that there was *Aspergillus* growing on the surface of the carpeting beneath the bed.

Why did this happen? Even though the tenant spent very little time in the apartment, many factors were involved. He kept the door and windows closed, so airflow in and out of the unit was at a minimum. It was a humid summer, and the air both inside the apartment and outside was laden with moisture. The carpeting in this apartment was laid directly on the "cool" concrete, which may have created dew point conditions. The tenant also took long hot showers in the morning and did not air out the unit. In addition, a downspout was creating puddles outside the building at the edge of the concrete slab.

To solve the problem, I recommended the management company install a dehumidifier in the unit, that the downspout be redirected away from the building, that the tenant air out the apartment after he took a shower, and that the wall-to-wall carpet be removed.

Wool Sensitivity

Wool is sheep hair. Human hair and sheep hair have similar structures in that each has an outer cuticle and an inner cortex. The cuticle consists of plates that look like a snake's scales wrapped around bundles of ropelike structures that give the hair its great tensile strength. "Split ends" of wool, like split ends of human hair, are the exposed bundles of cortex fibers. These ends have sharp points and may be responsible for the physical irritation caused by wool fabric.

Wool carpet hairs can become frizzy because of the physical abrasion of wear. The particulates (i.e., wool dander) that result from the breakup of the cuticle and cortex become airborne, sometimes in great numbers. One family had respiratory problems in the carpeted bedrooms on the second floor of their house but little trouble on the first floor, where there was oak flooring. The air in the bedrooms contained high concentrations of wool dander. The entire family moved into a hotel for a week while the wool carpeting was removed and wood floors were installed. When they went back home, their coughing did not recur.

Other Carpeting Concerns

Chemicals emitted from new wall-to-wall carpeting can be irritating. In most cases the odor disappears within a few days with no lasting negative effects. But sometimes carpets continue to off-gas for a long time; even the U.S. Environmental Protection Agency (EPA) had problems in its own offices with emissions from new carpeting.

One day I received a call from a woman who, after ten years of wearing her contact lenses with no difficulty, was experiencing eye irritation and had to revert to glasses. The irritation started shortly after she and her husband moved into their new home, which had wall-to-wall carpeting on every floor, and she insisted her eye problem was somehow related to the house. Her husband, a contractor who had designed and built the house as a gift to her, was deeply offended.

When I came to inspect the house, the couple answered my knock. The woman welcomed me warmly, but her husband was silent and seemed skeptical and hostile. Moments later, as I stood in the doorway, my eyes and lips started to burn. I detected the strong, characteristic odor of new carpeting. Perhaps you have noticed this smell in homes or stores. The odor has been attributed to 4-phenylcyclohexene (4-PC), a chemical in carpet backing made with styrene-butadiene plastic. Both the wife and I were affected by this or other chemicals, but the husband was not.

The carpeting in the basement was made with a different backing and had no 4-PC odor. After my visit, the husband and wife tried moving their bedroom from the second floor of the gracious twelve-room house into the partially finished basement, and all her symptoms went away. The husband was finally convinced that the upstairs carpet had caused a problem for his wife.

OFF-GASSING

Carpeting is only one of many materials that can off-gas irritating or annoying chemicals that cause headaches, hoarseness, and other symptoms in some sensitized individuals. Some vinyl-fiberglass screens, leveling compounds, and adhesives can also off-gas for weeks, months, or even years. Heat can intensify the off-gassing. I have a booth at the annual Old House Fair in Boston, sponsored by the Boston Preservation Alliance. One year I set up a vinyl-fiberglass screen (from my own storm door) with a very hot lamp shining on it to demonstrate off-gassing. A homeowner sniffed the screen and exclaimed, "That's the smell that's been driving me crazy in my house for the past three years!"

One homeowner who had built a large addition complained of a burned-plastic odor in her new workspace. She was about to replace her air conditioning system, but when we removed the vinyl-fiberglass insect screens from two skylights the odor disappeared.

Another woman called me because she wanted to eliminate a burning odor she had been noticing in her condominium for quite some time. She had just come home from the hospital with her newborn baby and was now concerned about the child's health as well. The other unit in the two-family building had recently converted from oil to gas heat, and she had already called in the gas company and fire department, to no avail. The man from the fire department, in fact, implied that she might be unbalanced and hysterical after pregnancy and childbirth.

She told me the smell was strongest in the late morning, and in the dining room. As soon as I arrived I smelled the acrid odor of heated vinyl-fiberglass insect screens. The screens were installed between the new storm windows and the old, leaky double-hung sash. The smell was strongest at the south-facing dining room wall, which started warming in the sun about 10 A.M. The owner told me the odor hadn't started until several months after the windows were installed, so at first she had a hard time believing the screens could be causing it, even though she immediately recognized the smell when she sniffed the air near the windows. Then she remembered that just before the odor began her neighbors had cut down two large trees that had been shading the dining room windows. The sun was now hitting that side of the building and the screens with greater intensity, heating the plastic and causing the odor. She replaced the vinyl with aluminum screening and then enjoyed the increased sunlight in her rooms without enduring the smell.

In a third case a couple was planning to move into a condominium with a spectacular view. An entire wall of living room windows faced the setting sun. Unfortunately the unit, which had been renovated three years earlier, was permeated by a peculiar smell that they found upsetting.

When I entered the apartment hall I noted a chemical odor not unlike one I had encountered in other homes, but more pungent. The sun's rays were very intense in the afternoon, and there was vinyl-fiberglass scrim (fine-mesh screen) to shade out the bright light. Suspecting the scrim was an odor emitter, I walked over to the windows and took a sniff. Indeed, the scrim had a peculiar chemical odor not unlike the one that had greeted me on entry.

The affable building manager, who had already spent hours trying to sort out this problem, offered to take away the scrim. He removed screws, anchors, and brackets and managed to eliminate all the offending scrim, at which point I noticed that the vinyl-fiberglass insect screens on the casement windows were also odor offenders. We removed these as well, and I recommended that the woman air out the apartment for several days.

Weeks later I received a call telling me a different odor was now present. This time the odor appeared to be coming from the carpeting. Since the couple had considered installing wood flooring anyway, they decided to eliminate the carpet. I was called back the day before the oak floor was supposed to be installed. With all the carpeting gone, the apartment reeked more strongly than ever with a new chemical odor, so much that I began to feel ill. Even though the insect screens, scrim, and carpeting were odor sources, it ultimately turned out that the biggest culprit was the polymer-containing leveling compound under the carpeting and pad.

In another case a man had a carpeted office space in the basement of his older home. An adjacent section of the basement had a dirt floor. The man developed serious respiratory distress and decided to move. He built a new house including a beautiful basement office with a private entrance at grade. Two years later he called and asked if I had any idea why he became so hoarse that he could barely speak whenever he spent a long time in his office. I went to his house and found that the air in the basement was quite irritating. The most likely source seemed to be the vinyl tile floor (he had avoided carpeting this time). The man still had an unused box of tiles, however, and these had no odor at all. I therefore suspected the floor adhesive was the culprit. I removed a tile from one of the closets and carried it upstairs, and he and I both took a sniff. That was it! Subsequent air testing revealed high concentrations of many chemicals from the adhesive, even though it had been applied months before. In this case the owner did nothing about the tile floor, which stopped off-gassing in about two years.

The best way to minimize chances of off-gassing like this is to spread a layer of the adhesive on a sample surface outside your home and let it dry for a few days (or weeks, if you have the time) before installing a new floor. If the smell lingers, find another adhesive.

Plastic Off-Gassing

A retired woman reported feeling ill from some odor whenever she read in front of her fireplace on cloudy days. The fireplace could have been a source of combustion gasses from the boiler in the basement, but it was tested repeatedly for carbon monoxide, and no gasses were ever found to be coming into the room. She and everyone involved in the original investigation suspected the weather might have something to do with the odor. The key, however, was her new reading lamp. On cloudy days she had to turn on the lamp to read her book. The plastic surrounding the threaded metal bulb socket was decomposing when the lamp was on, producing an odor that made her feel sick. In another home, the same burning odor appeared after living room table lamps were rewired.

Furniture Off-Gassing

New furniture made from medium-density fiberboard or particleboard can off-gas chemicals such as formaldehyde, which can irritate mucous membranes. The odor will usually dissipate in a matter of weeks or months, but occasionally furniture will continue to off-gas for over a year. I heard about a woman who purchased a new couch; shortly after putting it in her living room, she began to feel ill. The sicker she got, the longer she spent resting on her new couch. Doctors determined that she was sensitive to the formaldehyde emitted by the couch. She got rid of the piece and felt better.

If your new furniture has a lingering odor that is irritating, you might have to return it. Exposed fiberboard surfaces can be sealed to reduce off-gassing. If you have chemical sensitivities or react to formaldehyde, I suggest you buy furniture made from solid wood and be sure it is not coated with varnish containing urea formaldehyde.

FURNITURE WITH BIOLOGICAL CONTAMINATION

One woman called me because she noticed a strong odor of mold in the basement of a house she and her partner were considering buying. They had already had the home inspected, and the inspector had recommended they call me to see if I could help them find the source of the odor.

It was a warm summer day, and when I arrived all the windows were open. Were the owners too warm, or were they trying to air the place out? Despite the balmy temperatures, I felt quite a chill as the buyer and I walked in past the real estate agents and the owner. A $30,000 commission was in jeopardy, and my nose and microscope might stand in the way of the deal.

It was an older home, and the basement had a stone foundation. In one end was a couch in front of a television set; the sellers' children used this corner as a play area. There was a very strong mold odor at this end of the basement. I suspected the couch might be the culprit, so I tapped it and took a Burkard air sample of the dust cloud that rose from the surface. As if to deny that there was any problem, the real estate agent slumped noisily down onto the couch and relaxed into a comfortable position, commenting that she noticed no odor. When I looked at the air sample with a microscope, I found vast numbers of *Aspergillus* mold spores along with mite fecal pellets.

Ultimately my clients didn't buy the house, but not because of the odor. The floor sagged at the first-floor entry, and luckily there was a hole around a radiator pipe in the hall. I inserted my borescope to see if there was any moisture damage, but instead I found substantial structural decay from termites (termites too prefer damp spaces; see chapter 15).

Allergens accompany contaminated furniture. One asthmatic teenager was very proud of the couch in her bedroom because it changed the room into a sitting area. She spent many of her evening hours lounging on the couch, reading or chatting on the telephone with her friends. The shape of her body was pressed permanently into the cushions. Because her asthma could not be well controlled, her parents allowed nothing in the bedroom except her beloved couch, a dresser, and her bed. The room was spartan: there were no rugs on the floor, no curtains on the windows, no books on the shelves, and none of the bric-a-brac one would expect to find in a teenager's room. I pounded the couch cushion with my hand and took a brief Burkard air sample to collect the dust particles. I found that the sample contained many *Aspergillus* mold spores. When I talked to the parents, they immediately remembered that the couch had previously been used in the damp basement family room.

In another home a baby with serious mite and cat allergies was having asthma symptoms. The parents kept the baby's room scrupulously clean; the only furniture was a crib with a mattress covered in plastic and a cushioned chair for the nursing mother. My sample of the chair dust revealed long-forgotten secrets. The parents never realized that the nursing chair (a present from the baby's grandmother) had been stored for years in a cool, damp basement where Granny's cat spent long hours on hot summer days curled up on the chair. In consequence the cushion was contaminated with mold, mites, and dander. Every time the mother sat down to nurse her infant, a cloud of invisible airborne allergens surrounded the two of them.

Old chairs or sofas that have been stored in barns or basements may have been infested with small "insects" such as mites and spiders or small mammals such as mice. Antique bureaus may have mold growth, particularly in hard-to-see places like the bottoms of drawers or the furniture backing. Allergens in the dust can get shaken onto clothing when drawers are opened and closed.

My wife inherited a wooden coffee table from her parents. The piece had a cribbage board carved into its surface. It wasn't worth much, but she had fond memories of playing cribbage on it as a child. When she and her siblings grew up and moved away, her parents had stored the table in their barn. We set the table in front of our couch in the family room. The first time we played cribbage on it, I noticed an odor coming from the piece. I turned it over and found the bottom was completely covered with *Penicillium* mold. We went back to using our portable plastic cribbage set.

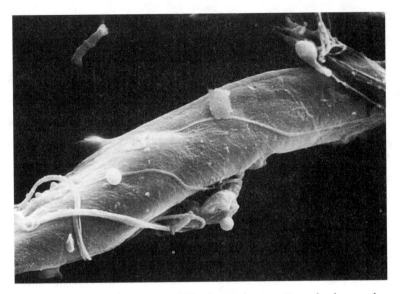

FIGURE 2.1. Cotton fiber with mold hyphae and spores. Even the dust on the saucer under a clay plant pot can become food for mold. Mold hyphae and growing mold were wrapped around this cotton fiber, which was in the layer of dust on the outside of the saucer. (1,500× SEM)

Cushioned items that have become moldy in basements should be discarded or disinfected and reupholstered. Hard-surfaced items covered with mildew can often be disinfected, then sealed with varnish or paint and used again.

PLANTS

Believe it or not, Christmas trees can be a source of mold or other allergens. They are cut long before they are sold and may be stored under damp conditions. Before purchasing a Christmas tree, look it over carefully to be sure it is not moldy. If anyone in your family or a frequent visitor is sensitive to mold, consider an artificial tree.

Many people like to keep plants in the house all year round, and in most cases they aren't a problem as long as the soil is kept free of moldy leaves and there is a moisture-proof barrier under the pot. But some people are careless. They give their indoor plants so much water that they might as well be using a garden hose. In one home I inspected, a plant had been watered carelessly and moisture had soaked into the living room carpet, creating a large stain. I found several species of mites living on the mold, moisture, and other nutrients in the stain. If a clay pot is sitting directly on carpeting, mold and mites can flourish because the water from the damp soil evaporates through the clay bottom.

Some plants should not be welcomed into the homes of allergy sufferers. One particular species, *Ficus benjamina* (weeping fig), has been associated with skin rashes and asthma symptoms. A report in an allergy journal theorized that irritating oils from this popular indoor plant soaked into the dust on the leaves, becoming airborne when the plant was disturbed. The patient described in the article felt relief from his allergy symptoms when the plant was removed. I had a client who experienced skin irritation whenever she even vacuumed near her *Ficus*.

PETS
Housebroken?

My mother-in-law always owned miniature dogs that she loved to distraction. She wasn't very successful in house-training her pets, though, and one dog in particular chose a corner of the living room for his "special spot." On rainy days, when the relative humidity was high, the entire room reeked. Obviously such areas are prone to mold growth and insect infestation.

One client in her seventies called me because after a life completely free of allergies she suddenly developed asthma. She had two enormous puppies that were not house-trained very well and often "made mistakes" on the white wall-to-wall carpeting. As a result she had to wash the carpeting "frequently." Unfortunately this resulted in repeated long exposure of nutrients (e.g., skin scales, dog waste) to moisture. The carpet was mold and bacteria heaven. When I sampled the air in the living room, I found that about 30 percent of the particulates were related to biological growth in the carpet.

One buyer was referred to me because he noticed a disturbing odor in the basement during his home inspection, after his offer on a house had been accepted. He was seriously considering walking away from the deal unless he could determine the cause and find a cure.

I parked in front of the enormous home and noticed that two dogs were frolicking in the fenced yard. The listing broker met me at the sidewalk and offered his opinion that perhaps the odor came from the automatic fragrance emitters that were spraying perfume into the basement air at regular intervals. I asked him to have the seller turn these off before I went in.

I met the buyer and his wife outside, and we all entered the grand sixty-year-old home, which had a completely finished basement. There was a basement billiards room with mahogany paneled walls and an oak parquet floor. On a shelf above the bar was a carton containing a dozen aerosol air freshener refills! When I shined a bright flashlight beam along the floor I could see that the oak strips were warped and swollen. The room reeked of animal urine. Numerous nail holes with oval black stains in the wood floor suggested that the floor had once been carpeted.

I checked the wood with a moisture meter, which measures resistance to the flow of electric current. The readings were off the scale. The resistance depends on the wood's moisture content: the wetter the wood, the less the resistance and the greater the electrical conductivity. Salt increases the conductivity as well and can make dry wood appear wet to the moisture meter. It was a wretchedly humid day, but the high meter readings were due not to moisture in the wood but to salts from animal urine. Outside, I explained to the buyer that the only way to completely get rid of the odor was to remove the antique flooring. It was a shame, for the wood was exquisite. If you own a dog, be sure the animal is completely housebroken.

Birds

One of my clients owned several birds that, though usually caged, were sometimes allowed to fly free in his carpeted home office. He became breathless one day after mild exercise, and his physician found he had hypersensitivity pneumonitis (a pulmonary disease; see the glossary). I took a Burkard air sample in the room and a second sample close to the bird as it flapped its wings. I found that the samples were nearly identical. There were numerous dander particles that appeared to be covered with a bacterialike organism.

In this case there were other conditions in his home (dirt crawl space, hot-air heating system, moldy basement) that may have contributed to his difficulties, but it's also true that several types of respiratory diseases are common to bird handlers.

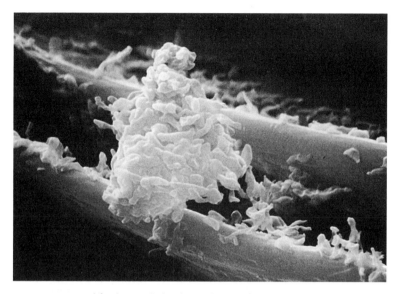

FIGURE 2.2. Bird feather with dander and microorganisms. A dander particle spans two strutlike structures from a cockatiel's wing feather. Note the bean-shaped organisms littering the feather surfaces and piled up in a cluster on the dander. In every home where cockatiels live, the air is filled with these organisms. Other birds probably produce similar bioaerosol. (4,000× SEM)

The Bad News

Most people who own beloved pets continue to keep the animals around even though the owners' eyes swell and their noses run. One parent of a little girl who was highly allergic to cats told me the family was very careful to keep the pet out of the child's bedroom. They did not realize this precaution would not protect the girl from exposure, because dander suspended in air moves with airflows throughout the house. (The dog and cat dander particles I observe in air samples look like pet skin scales, usually over 10 microns long. I am not certain whether they originate from the skin surface or hair follicles, but in either case the particles are probably covered with allergenic secretions from the sebaceous glands. Allergens in pet saliva from licking may also be present on pet fur and all fur dust.)

I give all people who have pet allergies the same bad news: try to find a new home for your animals. It's virtually impossible for someone who is allergic to a pet to share the house without some difficulty. Because they love their pets, many people are willing to suffer. But sniffling is one thing; asthma is another.

FRAGRANCE STINKS

I once saw a client of mine being interviewed on a television show about people who are bothered by scented products. One day while she was crossing the street to go to her physician's office, a car stopped in front of her. The window was open and the driver was drenched with aftershave. By the time she reached the doctor's office, she was wheezing.

One couple I worked with had three children who were experiencing chronic coughing in their impeccably maintained home. The parents had done almost everything they could to reduce allergens, including encasing mattresses and pillows in allergen control covers and installing hardwood floors in most of the rooms. After my first site visit, they had the contaminated ducts and air conditioning equipment cleaned and eliminated most of the remaining carpeting. The children continued to cough. On a subsequent visit I found that their mother was using detergent that contained fabric softener, fragrance, and enzymes. All the clothing and bedding in the house had the overpowering odor of this detergent; in addition, whenever anything was disturbed, bits of microscopic lint containing detergent residues became airborne.

After our first child was born, I began to wake up in the morning with irritated eyes. Within a few months my eyes would be swollen shut each morning. After a year or so the condition cleared up. When our second child was born I began to have the problem again. My wife finally figured out what was happening. When our children were infants, she added a liquid fabric softener to the wash to make their clothes fragrant and soft. Unfortunately she washed the babies' clothes with our own, and soon our shirts, pants, and sheets smelled like gardenias.

The aisles in supermarkets and drugstores are filled with perfumed potions: shampoos, conditioners, sprays, and gels for hair and lotions, creams, cologne, and aftershave for the skin, to name a few. Many people use fragrant room sprays and passive electric fragrance emitters to cover an odor rather than eliminating the source. Dishwashing liquids, floor and furniture polishes, tile cleaners, and laundry detergents also contain strong scents. Even products that are supposed to help allergy sufferers can cause problems. Several homeowners with asthma who sprinkled liberal amounts of a fragrant acaricide powder (a product for killing dust mites) on all the furniture and carpets were so irritated by the scent that they were forced to move out and hire professional cleaners to remove the chemical. After cautions issued by the EPA, the manufacturer voluntarily withdrew the product from the market.

Some companies are beginning to advertise "natural" products that supposedly are nontoxic but nonetheless contain fragrance. For asthma and allergy sufferers the issue goes beyond toxicity, however, because even "natural" scents can be irritating. The individual chemical constituents of both natural and synthetic fragrances have been tested on mice for sensory irritation. Many of the volatile organic compounds in fragrances affect the nervous and respiratory systems.

When I was teaching high school chemistry I used to pass around a small vial containing a chemical called cinnamaldehyde, the essential oil from cinnamon (and the odor of a popular pill-shaped red hard candy). The oil has a pleasing but pungent odor. One student became so enamored with the scent that she put a little on her skin, ignoring my warning not to touch the chemical. She immediately developed a brief rash. Amyl alcohol, a constituent of some liquors and fragrances, can also bother people. No matter how hard they try to resist, one good whiff of the vapors from the pure liquid will make them cough within twenty seconds.

Fragrances are so much a part of our landscape that we are often not even aware of them. Once you begin using fragrance-free products, you will be surprised at how much you notice scents. Our house is now fragrance-free, and whenever I am near anyone who uses a strongly scented shampoo, cologne, aftershave, or even deodorant, I not only am acutely aware of the perfume but, more often than not, find it irritates me. We all react with varying degrees to our environment. For those who have allergies and asthma or are chemically sensitive, heavy fragrances can exacerbate breathing difficulties and other reactions. I therefore recommend that people who are vulnerable use perfume-free products. In my opinion everyone should avoid using heavily scented products. Even if you aren't sensitive, someone who visits your home might be.

SMOKE GETS IN YOUR LUNGS

When health is at issue, it sometimes takes decades for the scientific community to recognize a danger. For example, lead was a common ingredient in gasoline, paint, and food cans until the second half of the twentieth century. Asbestos has finally been recognized as a carcinogen, but too late for pipe fitters and shipbuilders who were exposed to asbestos dust from insulation.

The public recognition that smoking causes lung cancer and heart disease is recent, within the past thirty to forty years. People still smoke, though, and exposure to secondhand smoke is also a serious concern. Cigarette smoke contains hundreds of known toxins, including formaldehyde, carbon monoxide, and hydrogen cyanide.

People sometimes call me because they are bothered by cigarette smoke in their apartments. Sometimes the odor comes from a smoker several floors below and is carried by hidden air currents within the building's structure. Very little can be done as long as the smoking continues. More often than not, I recommend that people with asthma symptoms caused by others' smoking either move or else convince their neighbors to quit the habit.

One of the cruelest things to do to a child with asthma is to smoke in the child's home. And even a person without asthma might be sensitive to cigarette smoke. If you, anyone you love, or anyone who lives in your house is sensitive to cigarette smoke or has asthma, it is essential that no one smoke there. In addition, if you have asthma, stay out of smoky bars.

RECOMMENDATIONS

CARPETING

- New carpeting should be allowed to off-gas either before installation or before you use the room. If you wonder whether new carpeting is off-gassing, take a clean fragrance-free paper towel, fold it in half twice, place it on a section of the rug, and cover it with aluminum foil. Secure the edges of the foil with removable tape. Leave this in place for twenty-four hours. Then quickly fold the paper inside the foil, take the package outside, and unwrap the foil just enough so you can take a sniff. If you detect the smell of new carpet, than the carpet is off-gassing.

- Synthetic rugs (polyolefin, nylon, and other synthetics) seem to bother some people less than wool rugs.
- Families with allergies or asthma should minimize wall-to-wall carpeting and rugs.
- If contaminated carpeting cannot be removed, cover it with a rug over a dust-impervious barrier.

FURNITURE

- Don't use furniture that has been stored in damp or moldy spaces (though wooden furniture that has gotten moldy can sometimes be disinfected, cleaned of all mold, and varnished inside and out to contain dust).
- Thoroughly clean used furniture, no matter what its value, before bringing such pieces into your home. If possible, avoid purchasing (or inheriting) used furniture with cushions.
- If you are sensitive to formaldehyde, avoid furniture made from medium-density fiberboard or particle board. If you suspect new furniture is off-gassing, use the foil test described above under carpeting.

PLANTS

- Pots should be set on moisture-proof barriers.
- Don't let dead leaves accumulate on the soil.
- Overhumidifying your home may make your plants happy, but it can promote biological growth.
- Consider an artificial Christmas tree.

PETS

- If you are allergic to your pet, find the animal a new home.

ODORS AND FRAGRANCES

- If you notice a chemical smell in a room, try to determine what's new in the room. Check window blinds, insect screens, any other plastic items (lamps, television sets, computer monitors), and new carpeting and padding in particular.
- If you are sensitized to heavy fragrances, avoid wearing perfume and cologne or even storing these substances in your home. Scented candles are romantic, but avoid them if they are irritating.
- If someone who lives in your home or spends a great deal of time there has allergies or asthma, avoid using perfumed products.

SMOKING

- There should be absolutely no smoking in the home of a person with asthma.

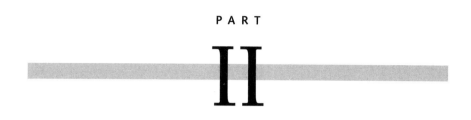

PART

II

Daily Life

3

Bedrooms

I am constantly amazed at the particulates I find in bedroom air. These particulates may make you cough when you get into bed, or they may make your asthma or allergy symptoms worse when you get up. In these circumstances many people feel they need to wash the sheets or blankets more frequently than usual. But you could spend your entire life cleaning floors, windows, shelves, and books, as well as laundering the bedspread, and you would still be coughing if the mattress or even one throw pillow was full of dust mites, mold, bacteria, or yeast. To solve the problem, the source of the irritating dust must be identified and eliminated.

MITES
Dust Mites in Our Beds

Mites grow and reproduce in spaces that are closest to our faces. Every time our body compresses the mattress or we crumple the pillow, air and dust particles from the stuffing are forced into the room. If the dust is contaminated, the expelled air carries with it particulates, such as mite fecal pellets, mold spores, yeast, or bacteria, that can cause respiratory distress.

Before I started looking at air quality problems, I had no idea how big a hazard dust mites can be. I found out when my eighth-grade son was hospitalized in the middle of the night with his first asthma attack. Even though we were always conscientious about changing sheets weekly and washing blankets and quilts every month, I decided to test all the beds in the house for mites. I vacuumed each mattress for several minutes, using a special filter on the nozzle that trapped all the dust and prevented it from going into the vacuum bag. I sent each filter full of dust to a laboratory for analysis. Fewer than 2 micrograms of mite allergens per gram of dust is considered low; over 10 is considered at significant risk for asthma. Each of our mattresses was outrageously high, with more than 30 micrograms of allergens per gram of dust. This is why I *always* recommend that people with allergies or asthma put dust mite allergen control covers on mattresses and pillows. These covers keep moisture and skin scales out and prevent existing allergens from escaping.

Encasing pillows and mattresses is one of the most important components of an allergy and asthma control strategy. If any family member has asthma or dust mite allergy, *all bed mattresses and pillows throughout the house should be encased.* It's not enough for people to cover the mattresses and pillows in the bedrooms, because dust mites can also flourish in couch pillows, the mattresses in sofa beds, and futon couches. I recommend that these too have allergen-control covers.

Some people think waterbeds can't harbor dust mites because the mattress is essentially a sealed plastic bag. It's true that mites cannot imbibe the moisture contained within the plastic, but the thick mattress pads used on water beds can contain a high level of mite allergens.

Down bedding can be a particular problem, for more than one reason. First, the species name for dust mite is *Dermatophagoides pteronyssinus*—Latin for "skin eating, feather loving." Thus anything that contains down can become a haven for mites. Second, the feathers themselves can break up into small sharp, airborne fibers that can be inhaled. The first time I saw down fragments under the microscope, I thought, "These could be irritants." I foolishly put my face into the sleeve of my parka, compressed the material, and inhaled. The pressure forced the down fragments into the air I breathed, and I coughed deeply and painfully for several hours.

One woman I know spent her winter holidays in a friend's basement apartment, sleeping in a guest bed that backed up against a brick wall. It was cold in the apartment, and she pulled the comforter over her face to keep warm as she slept. After her first night there she woke up with a mild rash on her face and neck. She applied soothing creams, but in the days that followed her skin turned red and mottled. In the last few days of her visit her chest felt tight. She and her friend thought the down comforter might be bothering her. As soon as she replaced the comforter with a cotton quilt, her rash faded and her chest discomfort subsided.

In another situation, two elderly sisters lived together. Every October the older sister began having respiratory symptoms. The younger sister always gave the older one her extra pillow so she would be more upright in bed to ease her coughing. This routine went on for years, until the older sister got worried about the increasing severity of her annual bouts with bronchitis. I found that her symptoms began each year when she put a down comforter on the bed as the weather turned cooler. She knew she was irritated by feathers, but she never realized that her own comforter was down because it was encased in a cotton cover. But there's more to the story: the pillow her sister lent her also was down filled! The cotton coverings did not prevent the release of irritants. Once she got rid of her down comforter and pillow, she also got rid of her bronchitis.

Sometimes in the air that comes from down, I find skin scales with holes in them. I often also find yeast and bacteria, which may be digesting the scales. Some of the skin scales are human. Others may be bird dander, so I have no idea whether some of these particulates were present when the bedding was new or whether they all appeared after long use. I do know, though, that whenever I find large numbers of these seemingly "digested" skin scales in the bedroom air where down bedding is present, I also find breathing problems.

In my experience, many people who cough when they go to bed or when they first get up find relief when they get rid of their down pillows or comforters. Wool can also be a problem, so I suggest using bedding made of cotton or synthetic materials.

Dust Mite Hitchhikers

Dust mites travel in our clothing, and their allergens are carried in air currents. A child can have a mite-free bed, but if she lies on her sibling's mite-ridden bed, her own bedding will soon become infested. In one home I had an Allergenco air sampler operating in the bedroom of a child who suffered from allergies. The family had taken great care to eliminate all sources of dust in the room, and the air contained almost no particulates of any kind. As the sampler continued cycling on and off, I opened the door to the parents' bedroom and began to move around the room, disturbing dust. I took a sample with a Burkard sampler and found that the air was contaminated with mold and mite fecal material. Particulates from the air in the parents' room eventually flowed into the hallway and then into the child's bedroom. After a while the dust samples the Allergenco sampler collected in the child's room contained allergens from the air in the parents' room. You may not necessarily sense particles, but be assured that they move around with airflows in a house just as odors do.

EXCESS MOISTURE

Bedrooms can become mold greenhouses if too much moisture is present. Moisture can be introduced in unexpected ways. For instance, one teenager with asthma went off to college and found herself relatively symptom-free. When she returned home on vacation and went to bed the first night, her asthma symptoms flared up. It might seem that the air in the entire house was contaminated or that the girl's symptoms were caused by emotional upheaval, but the truth is that during high school she had showered every night before going to bed, then placed her mop of wet hair directly on her pillow. The pillow she slept on at home for at least six hours each night was covered with mold.

The higher the relative humidity, the more accessible moisture is to mold and to microscopic insect life. Taking long showers in bathrooms next to bedrooms introduces water vapor into the indoor system. People who use humidifiers should monitor relative humidity with a hygrometer and maintain it below 35 percent during the winter. For homes near the shore, this is particularly important in carpeted bedrooms with concrete slab floors. In one family an infant suffered from bouts of wheezing, monthlong colds, and ear infections. In the baby's bedroom, barely visible colonies of pale yellow *Aspergillus* mildew grew on the bottoms of the dresser, bed, and table. (After gently waving a notebook to disturb dust, I found that the concentration of *Aspergillus* spores in the bedroom was thousands of times higher than in the outside air.) In warm, moist climates, you should keep the relative humidity below 60 percent with a dehumidifier or air conditioner.

One woman who constantly ran two steam humidifiers in her bedroom all winter started having severe allergy symptoms. The moisture had condensed on the cold exterior wall of the house. Behind the peeling wallpaper, I found the plaster completely black with mold. Dust hung like vines from the box spring beneath her bed, and when I looked at a sample of the dust with a microscope I found mites nibbling on the mold-covered dust balls. In the home of one client with a chronic cough and a diagnosed mold allergy, a bedroom humidifier ran all night during the winter. In the morning the couple left the bedroom door closed and lowered the thermostat before they went to work. Excessive relative humidity during the day allowed *Penicillium* to grow invisibly in the coarse cellulose on the bottom twelve inches of the grasscloth covering the cool outside walls.

Types of Room Humidifiers

There are four types of room humidifiers: steam, warm mist, ultrasonic, and evaporative pad. Some are more conducive to IAQ problems than others. I encourage people not to use ultrasonic or evaporative pad humidifiers. An ultrasonic humidifier, also known as a cool mist humidifier, uses sound energy to convert liquid water directly into microscopic droplets that are suspended in an air stream blowing through the unit. The trouble is that whatever minerals, bacteria, or algae are in the water to begin with can be aerosolized and distributed throughout the mist.

Most evaporative pad humidifiers contain an evaporative cellulose (paper) mesh pad. Water from the surface evaporates into air that is drawn across the material by the fan. I have seen the pads of several such humidifiers covered with mold and bacteria. In four homes the pads were black with potentially toxic *Stachybotrys* mold. This type of humidifier is prone to biological contamination for two reasons: first, the cellulose pad itself can serve as a nutrient; second, the mesh pad acts as a filter, capturing biodegradable particulates (such as skin scales and cornstarch from body powder) from the air. Since they are so prone to contamination, I believe humidifiers with cellulose evaporative pads should be banned. In one home a mother and her daughter had been suffering from continuous respiratory problems for most of the winter. The worse their symptoms became, the longer they operated their evaporative humidifier. I found very high levels of actinomycetes (filamentous bacteria) in the air and on the pad. The family stopped using the humidifier, cleaned up house dust, and within two weeks mother and daughter were well again.

Steam humidifiers and warm mist units both boil water, and they emit only water vapor; minerals and other contaminants remain behind in the water reservoir. In a warm mist humidifier the "steam" is mixed with and cooled by room air before the vapor leaves the unit. A warm mist humidifier is also equipped with a humidistat, which shuts it off when the humidity in the room reaches the set value. (Old-fashioned steam humidifiers do not have any type of control; they just make steam (until the water runs out), so they can introduce excess moisture into the room.)

Of all the types of room humidifiers available, I recommend a warm mist unit. Remember to keep children away because of the warm vapor and the small reservoir of boiling water. Regardless of the type of humidifier you have,

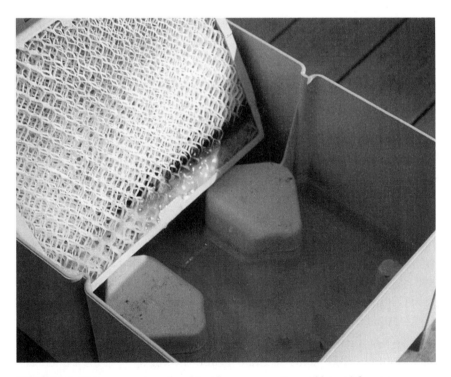

FIGURE 3.1. Water reservoir and pad inside an evaporative pad humidifier. A teenager suffered asthma symptoms in a room where this evaporative pad humidifier was running. Biological growth covered the bottom of the pad (called a water-wicking filter) where it was submerged in water. A black band of *Stachybotrys* mold flourished at the waterline.

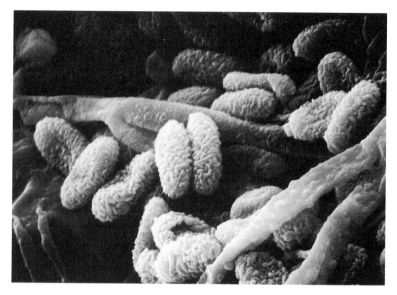

FIGURE 3.2. *Stachybotrys* spores and hyphae growing along the surface of a cellulose pad from an evaporative pad humidifier. A tape sample taken at the bottom of the humidifier pad was covered with *Stachybotrys* mold spores and hyphae. Dust from the top of the humidifier also contained *Stachybotrys* spores, suggesting that the spores were ejected from the pad when the humidifier blower operated. (2,500× SEM)

you should monitor the relative humidity with a hygrometer, available in most hardware stores.

BEDROOM "GUESTS"

One day I received a call from a retired professional. Although he had never had any allergies before, now he was wheezing and sniffling and could no longer enjoy his new leisure life. Occasionally his symptoms even appeared at his favorite seafood restaurant; once when he was eating there with friends, his nose ran so much that he had to make his embarrassed apologies and leave before the meal was finished. He had even been told to see a psychiatrist because his nose started to run whenever he entered two specific areas in his home.

There were tropical fish tanks in both his home and the restaurant. The tank in his den at home had a black plastic cover with a hinged access panel so he could feed the fish. I lifted the cover and saw a layer of fine brown "dust" adhering to the underside. I took a sticky tape sample and looked at the dust with my microscope. Dust mites were there, wriggling and stuck to the tape, but the brown dust consisted almost entirely of damp mite fecal pellets that were being digested by bacteria.

When the man threw flakes of fish food into the water, some of them stuck to the damp underside of the opened cover. It's not surprising that I found this microcosm, since fish food is as appealing to dust mites as skin scales. In laboratories, dust mite colonies are fed these high-protein flakes.

I didn't find a lot of whole dust mite fecal pellets in the air in the room, but I did find fragments of pellets, as well as clumps of bacteria and small bits of partially digested skin scales. I suspect some of these particulates were allergens. The irony is that sometimes the only pets people with asthma can have are fish, and in this case a fish tank was a source of allergens.

Fish tanks are favorite items in children's bedrooms, and it's not only dust mites that are a concern. Sometimes a filter placed on the outside leaks onto shelves, walls, and floors. One unfortunate youngster was enthusiastic about feeding his fish, and he often spilled fish food on the floor near the tank. Water from a leaking exterior filter dripped onto the food flakes, and mold soon proliferated in the carpet. Another tank's leaking filter led to mold's destroying volumes M, N, and O of an encyclopedia on the shelf below the aquarium. Filtration and aeration systems placed inside the fish tank can also cause problems: they bubble air through the water, and when the bubbles break, algae and other bioaerosols are dispersed into the room air.

Children also keep rabbits and hamsters in their rooms. These animals shed dander and fur. Some people sleep with cats and dogs, which are living dust mops. One boy who slept with his cat every night woke each morning with a rash on his face. The parents figured out the source of the irritation only when they realized that the family cat spent much of the day sleeping on exposed fiberglass insulation in the basement ceiling. Fiberglass fibers often have sharp ends, like broken glass. When the boy slept with his face next to the cuddly pet, his skin was irritated by the insulation fibers stuck to its fur. In another home, I found basement mold and dander from the family's cat in dust taken from their dog's fur.

Animals don't have to be alive to carry contaminants. Stuffed animals can be full of mites and dander if they are in the bed and thus serve as miniature pillows. The filling of even new stuffed animals can be allergenic. Two cases in the medical literature describe children whose asthma was made worse by beanbag toys. One of the toys was filled with crushed walnut shells, not beans, and the other was filled with soybeans; in each case the child was sensitized to the stuffing.

CLOSETS

Cedar walls or mothballs in bedroom closets emit chemicals that can irritate people who are sensitized to them. In addition, most mothballs are pesticides (either napthalene or p-dichlorobenzene), which can be harmful to anyone's health. An ordinary closet can be a source of mold and mite contamination, particularly if it is in a shaded outside corner of the house or is cantilevered (overhanging an exterior wall). The temperature of such an outside wall may be below the dew point, causing condensation to form. Mildew and mites find a welcome home in such locations. If the relative humidity is high enough, mildew can spread to shoes, clothing, stored boxes, and carpeting. As people remove their clothing and shake it, irritants become airborne and flow into the bedroom.

A physician referred a patient to me who was having difficulty controlling his asthma symptoms, which occurred wherever he went. I found mold growing in his closet and mite fecal pellets in his clothing, including the jacket he wore to work. I too had an experience with contaminated clothing. I purchased an expensive wool jacket in a fine clothing store. The first time I put it on, I started coughing and wheezing. I decided to return it, thinking the wool was bothering me, but I decided to investigate first. I put the jacket in a plastic bag, beat the bag, and collected the aerosolized particulates with a Burkard sampler. I was surprised to find no wool dander particulates, but I was astonished to see mite fecal pellets and mold spores in the dust from the wool. Most likely someone had bought the jacket before me, taken it home to a wretchedly contaminated closet, then returned it to the store. I had the "new" jacket dry-cleaned and was able to wear it after that without any ill effects.

CONDITIONING THE AIR

People often use window air conditioners to control the air in their bedrooms. Air conditioners increase our comfort by cooling air and removing moisture,

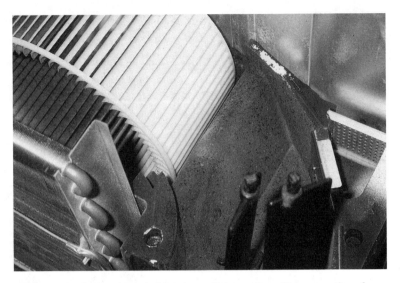

FIGURE 3.3. Blower on a window air conditioner. One client experienced asthma symptoms whenever the air conditioner was turned on. When the unit was removed from its metal case, we could see that the interior sides of the white blower blades were black with mold. Mold colonies were also growing in the dust on other plastic surfaces within. Microscopic examination revealed that the contaminants consisted entirely of *Cladosporium*.

but because nearly all air conditioners have inadequate dust filters, biodegradable material accumulates on the cold, damp cooling coils. Within days, mold, bacteria, or yeast can start to grow in the dust on the coils. In dirty air conditioners the mold can spread to the interior walls of the unit and even to the blower, growing until every speck of dust is consumed and converted to hyphae and spores. The air movement from the blower may then circulate these organisms. Even if the organisms themselves aren't circulating, the odors they produce fill the air inside the unit and pass into the room with airflows, alerting people that an indoor air quality problem is brewing.

All types of dust should be kept off air conditioner coils because of the very high likelihood of biological growth. Unfortunately, no manufacturer I know of makes a proper filter for a window or wall air conditioner. You have to buy the highest quality filtering material you can find and cut it to fit (see chapter 10). Be certain the filtering material does not touch the wet coil or it will soak up water and become moldy. Also be sure the perimeter of the filter fits tightly, to prevent dust from bypassing the filter. The filter should not be used for more than one season. I do not recommend using a washable filter; like a dirty sponge, it can never be cleaned.

Some people leave window air conditioners in place for years. This is asking for trouble. If you find that running your air conditioner makes your allergy or asthma symptoms worse, have the unit cleaned and disinfected. In fact, if you have allergies or asthma, window air conditioners should be removed and cleaned and disinfected at the beginning of every cooling season.

Sometimes window air conditioners and wall heat pumps (which cool air and also provide heating) can create excessive indoor moisture. I inspected a new condominium in a large building in which sections of the wood floor in nearly every room had to be replaced. The heat pump wall units were tipped improperly, and water from condensation dripped to the inside rather than the outside, warping the wood floors. In one home a child developed asthma symptoms because the water from a window air conditioner dripped onto the carpet under his desk, causing mold growth. As he sat at his desk to do his homework, his feet disturbed the moldy dust in the carpet fibers and he breathed in the spores.

Because we spend so much time in our bedrooms, controlling the quality of the air there is essential for maintaining health. In families with allergies or asthma, it is vital.

RECOMMENDATIONS

THE BED

- Use allergen-control covers on *all* pillows and mattresses in the house. Cover the mattresses on sofa beds and futon couches as well.
- Wash sheets weekly in hot water.
- Wash blankets at least monthly and tumble weekly in a warm or hot dryer for about twenty minutes.

- Wash quilts monthly and be sure to dry them thoroughly. Tumble weekly in a warm or hot dryer for at least twenty minutes.
- If you do not need to encase pillows, tumble them at least monthly in the dryer and replace them periodically.
- Wash and thoroughly dry mattress pads weekly.
- If a friend offers you a mattress, refuse it with thanks. Secondhand mattresses may be contaminated with mites.
- Avoid down quilts or pillows.
- If you are sensitized, avoid using wool on beds.
- Don't overload beds with pillows and stuffed animals.
- Stuffed animals that you can't part with can be tumbled in the dryer weekly.

EXCESSIVE MOISTURE

- Don't go to bed with wet hair or clothing.
- If you use a humidifier, monitor the relative humidity with a hygrometer (sold in most hardware stores). Keep humidity below 40 percent in the winter (preferably closer to 35 percent).
- Follow the manufacturer's directions about cleaning and maintaining humidifiers. Do not use evaporative pad or ultrasonic models. I recommend using only warm mist humidifiers.

PETS

- Keep dogs, cats, rabbits, hamsters, and other pets out of your bedroom.
- People with asthma should not have fish tanks in their bedrooms.
- People who own pets should not lie on the bed of anyone who has asthma or allergies.

CLOSETS

- If the odor of a bedroom cedar closet bothers you, either remove the cedar or seal the walls with aluminum foil.

- Keep your closet as clean and dust-free as the rest of the bedroom.
- Don't store items against outside walls in closets or directly on the floor if there is concrete under the carpet.

CLOTHING

- Wash or dry-clean clothing frequently.
- Frequently worn but rarely cleaned items of heavy clothing such as winter jackets and coats should be tumbled periodically in a warm or hot dryer.
- Dry cleaning kills mites and destroys some mite allergens.

AIR CONDITIONERS

- Keep window air conditioners clean by having them professionally washed and disinfected annually; to accomplish this, exterior cases have to be removed.
- Install the best filtering material you can buy that is compatible with your unit. If you can see through an air conditioning filter, it is inadequate.
- The filter should be installed so no unfiltered air gets onto the cooling coil and so it is not in contact with the coil.
- Filters should be changed each season.
- Be sure no water from the window air conditioner (or wall heat pump) drips to the inside.

MISCELLANEOUS

- Use a a bright light and mirror to check for mildew under furniture.
- Avoid using wall-to-wall carpeting in bedrooms; use small washable rugs instead.
- I do not recommend using mothballs or pesticide sprays inside the house, especially in the bedroom.

4

Bathrooms

A bathroom is usually one of the smallest rooms in a house yet one of the most intensively used. Because water is always present, you must pay particularly close attention to potential sources of indoor air quality problems.

TOILETS
The Hot Seat

Using warm water to flush a toilet may sound wasteful, but sometimes it's not a bad idea. In moist climates or on humid days, the cold toilet tank and connecting pipes may be below the dew point so that moisture from the air condenses on them and drips onto the floor or rug, where odor-causing mold and bacteria can flourish. Piping some hot water into the tank can keep it above the dew point and prevent condensation. On the other hand, too much hot water can create a different problem.

One cold winter day, during a prepurchase inspection of a "three family" home, I discovered an illegal basement apartment—one large room functioning as kitchen, living room, bedroom, and bathroom. The kitchen area was on a raised wood platform, and at the end of the L-shaped kitchen counter was a toilet. Although this clearly was the kitchen of an immodest chef, two even more peculiar conditions immediately caught my eye. In the foreground, I could see smoke coming out of the chimney pipe connector on the building's oil furnace. The furnace exhaust was supposed to be going into the chimney, but the pipe had been disconnected so the exhaust gases would keep the unit warm. In the background, smoke was coming out of the toilet bowl.

It was a scene from hell—and smelled like it. The "apartment" reeked of burning oil. It was hard to believe someone lived there. Had the combustion gases from the furnace contained carbon monoxide, the tenant wouldn't have been *living* there very long.

The "smoke" from the toilet turned out to be steam, which is formed when liquid water is heated and evaporates as vapor. When the vapor hits the colder air, it condenses into droplets that remain suspended. You can't see water vapor in the air, even though it is there all the time, because it is a gas and just mixes invisibly with the other gases in air. You can see steam droplets, however, because they reflect light. When the droplets evaporate they become vapor again and disappear from view.

Apparently whoever "renovated" the basement had set the water heater's thermostat to "scald" and inadvertently (unless he was hoping for a second source of heat) attached the toilet tank to the hot water rather than to the cold water. The flush lever was stuck and the tank's flapper valve was open, so boiling hot water was running continuously into the bowl. Steam was billowing from the toilet bowl into the cold basement air.

The Wax Ring

A toilet bowl is usually secured to the floor by two bolts. If the floor isn't perfectly flat, or if there is too much or too little space between the toilet bowl and the sewer pipe flange, the toilet may rock. A wax ring under the toilet creates the watertight seal between the toilet and the sewer pipe. This ring is all that keeps flushed water in the piping. If a toilet moves from side to side at all, the seal is broken and water can leak out, soaking into the floor around the toilet and dripping onto the ceiling below to produce a circular stain with mold. If there is a bathroom rug, the water produces an environment where mold can grow. If the situation gets bad enough, the toilet can start to tip as the wood under it decays. If the wood rots so much that the floor gives way, the pipe underneath it may not be strong enough to support the toilet. If your toilet is tipping like this, repair it before you find yourself sitting on the throne in your living room!

A disrupted wax ring seal also lets sewer gas enter the room—a most un-pleasant smell. Even if you can barely detect the gas, it can cause nausea and headaches. The source of sewer gas is often difficult to locate, since the emis-sion can be intermittent. The flow of sewer gas out of a pipe depends on the difference in pressure between the gases inside the pipe and the air in the room, which in turn depends on pressure differences between the air in the pipe and the outside air. The sewer system of the house is vented to the outside by an open-ended pipe at the roof called a stack. When the wind blows it changes the air pressure in both the stack pipe and the house, and the rela-tion between the two can fluctuate. Air always flows from spaces with higher pressure to those with lower pressure, so if the pressure of the pipe gases is higher, sewer gas will blow into the room. (On particularly windy days, the water level in the toilet bowl can fluctuate erratically as the wind blows over the stack and pressure in the drainpipe system changes.) A TIF 8800 com-bustible gas detector, available from some catalog instrument suppliers (see the resource guide at the end of the book), is often useful to pinpoint sewer gas emissions.

If you have a loose toilet, a wax seal that isn't airtight is the most likely source of sewer gas. In older homes, however, there may be a broken or open vent pipe in a wall. One client removed the garage roof and demolished a room in her house before discovering that the source of a sickening odor was a bro-ken vent pipe leaking sewer gas into the bathroom wall.

THE SINK

Common sources of water leaks in sinks are worn valve packings (the seal around the stem for the hot and cold water valve handles) and leaks around the base of the faucet. Water leaking into the vanity below can cause rot and odor. Some vanities are packed so full of bottles that a leak at the sink trap or pop-up lever arm escapes notice. To check for leaks, lower the pop-up, fill the sink with water and drain it, then look underneath with a flashlight and mirror.

Even small amounts of water, if continually applied, can rot a finished wood floor or other wood surface. For example, a vanity should be flush with the back wall and installed with a watertight backsplash; otherwise water may drip down the back, rotting the wall and the vanity. In addition, if a vanity is installed almost flush with the bathtub or close to it, you won't be able to see water dripping from a tub or shower. When kept consistently damp, these vanities can decay and be a source of mold odor. If the mold is disturbed, spores will become airborne.

A whole forest of mold can be flourishing beneath your sink or at the side of your vanity. Although you may not always see the mold, you will most likely smell it. Odorous biological growth also finds a home in sinks without vanities. Occasionally a very annoying moldy odor will come from the sink, particularly an older wall-hung model. This is the result of microbiological decay of nutrients such as soap and dust in the overflow; you can treat this condition with diluted bleach.

THE SHOWER AND TUB

When using a shower curtain, be sure all the water stays inside the tub or shower enclosure. Sometimes it helps to watch when someone else takes a shower so you can see where the water is dripping or spraying out. Even small leaks can cause problems. If the floor is tile, the water will probably evaporate. Water can leak underneath tile, though, if there is loose caulking or grout. Soon the tile will loosen, and the situation will get worse. Water can also pool under curled linoleum edges and rot the subfloor beneath. Push on the flooring near a tub to see if there's decay below; if the floor bends (or your finger goes through), you have a problem.

In one apartment a simple grout crack led to long-term concealed leakage of shower water under a tub. This leak had serious health consequences, for the water soaked into the plywood subfloor under the wall framing and spread to the adjacent bedroom of an asthmatic child. For months the carpeting in the room had been secretly soaking up the daily deluge. The moisture led to the growth of *Aspergillus* mold in the subfloor, pad, and carpet dust, and mites and other insects flourished. Unfortunately the child played in this corner of her bedroom; she wheezed when she breathed the spores and mite fecal material that aerosolized as she jumped on the carpet.

One day I received the kind of call all home inspectors dread, from a man whose house I had inspected. He was concerned about what he thought was water leaking from a bathroom pipe in the ceiling above the living room. The water had dripped onto a family heirloom—a harpsichord—and damaged the

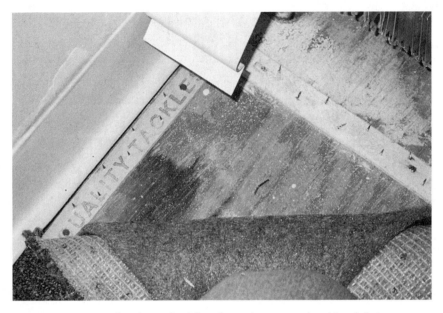

FIGURE 4.1. Stain in the plywood subfloor beneath carpet and pad in a baby's room. When the carpet and padding were peeled back in the corner of the bedroom of an asthmatic child, two signs of water leakage were visible. The nailheads holding the tack strip down were rusted, and the subfloor was water stained (the dark area beside the word "quality") and moldy. In addition, moisture had caused paint to bubble in a small area of the wall above the cove molding.

instrument's finish. His tone suggested that I should have known something was wrong with the pipe. It was a sticky situation, and to add to the tension, he was an attorney.

I went over there the next morning. The attorney led me to the harpsichord and pointed indignantly to a small discolored ring where water had landed. I looked up at the ceiling, and there was a pendant drop. Next we went upstairs to the bathroom. On the wall next to the tub was a wood baseboard. In the corner where the baseboard met the tub wall the tile floor looked dry, but when I tested the baseboard with my Tramex moisture meter, I obtained a damp reading. There was a slight crack in the paint film between the wall and the baseboard near the tub, suggesting that the wood along that intersection had at one time been swollen with water and had shrunk again while drying, separating the baseboard from the wall. I asked the man if he had just showered and then wiped up water in that corner. He hesitated momentarily and then said yes.

What had happened here? It seemed that when the man showered he did not always close the shower curtain completely at that end of the tub. Water ran down the wall at the end of the bathtub until it came to the flat top of the baseboard. Once the crack opened, the water flowed into it, down behind the trim and into the living room ceiling, then dripped onto the harpsichord. I recommended that he caulk into place a small triangular piece of plastic (a tub splash guard) made to prevent water from flowing over the wall edge of a tub, and I left his home feeling better than when I had arrived.

Shower curtains, even when properly used to keep water inside a tub or shower area, can become covered with biological growth, especially at the bottom edges, and become a source of odor. Shower curtains should be replaced periodically, particularly if they don't have adequate time to dry or if they start to smell. I recommend using an inexpensive shower liner that can be discarded and replaced when it gets discolored with growth.

Many people prefer shower doors, but these too must be kept clean. They can accumulate malodorous slime in the tracks—not easily removed! The frame must also be watertight. If caulk is not properly placed at the time of installation, as well as between the metal track and the tub's porcelain, water can leak out. In addition, when the shower door frame is installed, the vertex of the angle (where the ends of the vertical and horizontal pieces meet) must be embedded in caulk, for water pools at the ends of the lower track. Putting caulk at the inside of the corner or at the edge of the frame after it has been put in place will not provide a sufficiently watertight seal.

When my wife and I purchased our home, the seller mentioned at the closing that her family didn't use the shower in the third-floor bathroom much because the kids had more fun in the tub. The tub enclosure had sliding glass doors. Our fifteen-year-old daughter preferred to take showers—long and hot! One day my wife noticed a spreading ceiling stain in the hallway beneath the bathroom.

She ran up the stairs and shouted through the door, "Turn off the shower!" When I looked closely at the tub, I found that the lower corner of the shower door track was caulked only on the inside. In fact the frame was loose, and water from the shower was sneaking out over the edge of the tub, draining down through the joint between the tub and the tile floor, and pooling on the ceiling beneath. To stop the leak, I removed all four pieces of the metal frame and caulked the wall and tub sections back into place. I also caulked the floor joint.

Sometimes even the best shower curtain or door won't prevent water from escaping because people are careless once they've finished showering. We had a houseguest one summer who insisted on stepping out of the tub soaking wet and dripping on the cloth bathroom rug. In addition, she left the bathroom door closed for the rest of the day. This became a little tug of war between us; I would open the door whenever I could, and she would close it. She felt it was impolite to leave a bathroom door open even if no one was inside.

Within two weeks the entire third floor of the house began to reek from the bacteria growing on the wet nutrients in the bathroom rug. The sour smell reminded me of an old dirty sponge. Wet towels can also acquire that smell if they don't dry out fast enough, so it's always a good idea to hang towels to dry, preferably outside the bathroom during humid weather. But bacteria can cause more than odors. One client wheezed in his house, especially in the bathroom. On the tile floor next to the tub was a small cloth bath mat. He told me he washed it regularly, yet I found that the material was severely contaminated with bacteria. Whenever he stepped onto the rug, particulates (digested skin scales, bacteria) became airborne and from there settled with other dust onto bathroom surfaces. The client's wheezing subsided after the bath mat and all the wall and floor room dust were eliminated.

Water Ways

Water can escape a tub or shower from any side. In an older home, windows inside a tub or shower enclosure can cause a particular problem, especially where a tub on legs has been replaced by a built-in tub with shower. It is extremely important to cover such windows adequately with waterproof curtains to protect them from the shower water, or the windowsill and even the entire wall can rot.

After showering, however, leave this kind of window uncovered to allow for drying. Windows within tub and shower enclosures, as well as shower doors, should be glazed with safety glass in case someone slips and falls against them. Safety glass shatters into many small fragments, whereas normal plate glass breaks into long, sharp shards.

On winter days I have seen icicles coming out of exterior walls under bathroom windows. At one home inspection I suspected concealed wall decay behind asphalt siding, and I recommended the buyer have the siding removed near the bathroom window before signing a contract to purchase the house. The carpenter he hired found that underneath and to the right and the left of the windowsill, the wood siding and the wall structure behind it had been turned to dust by fungal growth. Even if you replace an old wooden sash window with a vinyl one, the wood structure is still vulnerable to water that may leak around the window frame.

We must try to control water, the essential "ingredient" of bathrooms, but it has a mind of its own. It can seep insidiously behind loosened wall tile in the tub enclosure or leak intermittently from the tub overflow (the opening in the metal escutcheon plate around the pop-up control below the faucet). If the overflow seal is ineffective but only a small amount of water leaks past, you may have only paint blisters or a minor stain on the ceiling beneath the tub. Damage can be substantial, however, if someone fills the tub to the level of the plate and then climbs in.

How can you avoid a tub overflow disaster in your home? Check the escutcheon plate; it should not move at all. If the plate is loose, don't fill the tub to the level of the plate, because the water will rise when you get in the tub, and water will overflow. Have the plate fixed; and remember, just tightening the two plate screws may not be adequate if the seal ring is broken or out of position.

Indoor Rain

You may notice after you take a shower that water condenses on the mirror (turns from vapor to liquid state). In fact, water condenses on all surfaces in a bathroom, particularly on cold surfaces such as exterior walls, uninsulated ceilings, and windows. Accumulations of water on wooden window sashes can lead to wood decay by mold. After someone takes a shower, the shower curtain or doors should be left partially open to allow airflow to evaporate the water remaining on the tub or shower walls. Most bathroom exhaust fans do not create sufficient airflow to remove all the moisture in the air and on the walls, so I also recommend that people leave the bathroom door open after a shower. (The water that evaporates from a bathroom increases the amount of vapor in the house air and thus raises the dew point.)

One couple who called me had decided to rent an apartment from the young man's parents. He had asthma, and his girlfriend was an attorney. During the first winter they noticed mold growing on the walls of the apartment—worst in the outside-corner closet, but also on the wall next to their bed.

They washed clothing in the bathtub and hung it on the shower curtain rod to dry. They took long, hot showers. During the day, since both worked, they turned down the thermostats on the baseboard electric heaters to save money. (As it turned out, this was penny wise and pound foolish.) They also kept the shades pulled down on the new insulated-glass wooden sash windows. The shades kept the heated air away from the windows, so they stayed cooler than the rest of the air in the apartment (which wasn't that warm to begin with!). The window glass was below the dew point of the apartment air, and moisture from the interior living and laundering then condensed on the new windows. Before long the window rails, which sat submerged under condensed moisture, began to rot. The father's ire was roused, the son's asthma flared, and the young lady's legal instincts sought someone to fault for the moldy clothing she had to discard from her closet.

Unwelcome Decoration

The most common complaint I hear about bathrooms is that there is mold growing on the ceiling. Warm, moist air from showering is less dense than the air around it, so it rises to the ceiling, where water condenses on the cooler surface. To minimize condensation, be sure there is adequate insulation above the bathroom ceiling. If you can't retrofit insulation, it may be easier to install sheet foam insulation and a new drywall ceiling. If mildew grows on the walls, insulate them as well.

Mold also can grow on tub and shower tile grout, on wall surfaces, and in rugs. Given a damp environment, biological growth can flourish on just about anything organic, including skin scales, soap film, dust from cornstarch body powder, cellulose or glue from wallpaper, caulk, and the resins in paints.

One way to prevent the growth of mold and bacteria, in addition to controlling moisture, is to limit potential nutrients by keeping dust at a minimum.

One condominium owner was plagued by dust in her home, which she thought came from a year-long renovation project in the unit above hers. She said the dust deposits were heaviest in the bathroom. She wanted to sue the condominium association, and she called me to help her gather evidence for her case. When I examined the bathroom air sample with a microscope, I discovered that the dust contained mostly cornstarch and short, fibrous cellulose lint. It's easy to guess that the cornstarch came from body powder, but where do you think the lint came from? Toilet paper shreds. My advice? Forget the lawsuit, tear the toilet paper only at the perforations, and buy body powder made from talc, not cornstarch (and use sparingly).

Any floor heat or air conditioning supply can accumulate dust. In areas prone to moisture, such as the bathroom, the dust can become moldy, particularly if the supply duct is in a cold attic, basement, or crawl space. In one home the cornstarch on a wall register got damp and moldy, and when the heat was on spores blew into the bathroom.

Mold that is growing on a bathroom heat or air conditioning supply register can be a significant risk to someone who is sensitized. But is the mold you see on the ceiling or on the tile grout a health risk? The danger depends on the number of spores you breathe in. Surprisingly, mold that is growing on the ceiling may not cause a problem because the spores do not regularly become airborne. (Once I made the mistake of taking an air sample in a bathroom after disturbing the ceiling mold; there were thousands of spores in the air sample!) The type of black mold that often discolors grout grows mostly beneath the surface of the material, and the spores do not readily become airborne. Just the same, because mold can be a source of odor and spores, I recommend that people disinfect the bathroom ceiling and tile grout with diluted bleach.

Another way to limit mold and bacterial growth is to lower moisture levels. There is always lots of moisture in bathrooms, for obvious reasons, but inadequate ventilation makes the situation worse. If the excessive moisture is a long-standing condition, biological growth is more apt to occur. Keep your bathroom clean and dry, and both you and the room will benefit.

Drying Out

After showering, keep the bathroom door and shower open. If mildew develops, use a small fan to circulate bathroom air and further speed evaporation. Keep the fan where it can't be knocked over easily, and plug it into an outlet protected by a ground fault interrupt (GFI). (Don't use a fan before you disinfect a surface with existing mold, lest you stir up spores.)

Building codes require at least a window or exhaust fan in every bathroom, to reduce moisture and odors. In most cases this means having separate ducts to the exterior for each fan. In one condominium this was not the case. The owner was complaining about fabric softener odors and lint in the bathroom. The bathroom exhaust shared a hose with the dryer exhaust. When the dryer was operating, it vented into the bathroom, because the hose between the bathroom and dryer was shorter than the distance between the dryer and the outside. There was thus less resistance to the airflow from the dryer to the bathroom than from the dryer to the exterior. To solve the problem, the owners installed a separate vent hose for the dryer.

Another of my clients who had allergies noticed that whenever he was in the bathroom and the exhaust fan was turned off, he began to cough. Why did this happen? This bathroom was on the first floor. Warm air rises, and in the winter warm house air leaked out (exfiltrated) from the uppermost levels. Cold air infiltrated at the lowest levels to replace the air that had leaked out. In this bathroom the seal at the vent kit (the outside end) of the exhaust hose was not airtight (few are), so when the exhaust fan was turned off cold air leaked through the exhaust hose into the room. Since the inside of the hose was at a lower temperature than the moist air passing through it from the bathroom when the exhaust fan was on, condensation occurred inside the hose, and mold grew on the dust inside. Air continued to enter the house through the mold-lined hose, carrying spores with it.

In the end my client disconnected the exhaust fan and no longer coughed when he was in the bathroom. Instead he installed a window, which ventilated the room just fine. If you have an exhaust, check the vent to be sure the damper opens when the fan turns on and closes when the fan is off. I also recommend an exhaust with a squirrel-cage blower rather than a propeller fan, since it has greater capacity.

UNHEALTHY CLOUDS

We think of water as a transparent fluid (unless it contains particles that reflect or absorb light). Now and then you might find bits of rust or minerals from the tap in your glass, so you throw out the water and draw a fresh glass. But water, whether it is piped into your home or bottled, comes from an ecological system that contains living things like fish, plants, snails, and insects. If the water is from a reservoir, pigeons, geese, and other birds may fly overhead, and ducks, dogs, or even people may enjoy a swim. All these living things periodically leave their "signatures" in the water.

Water and air are both fluids and are mixed by a cyclic movement called convection. For example, air warmed by a light bulb will rise to the ceiling and flow toward the walls, pushing the cooler air in front of it down the walls toward the floor. Similarly, in a lake or reservoir, warmer water floats to the surface and cooler water sinks. In the fall the air above the surface cools, causing the top layer of water to cool as well. As the water cools it sinks, creating a gentle turbulence.

When water is stratified or layered by temperature, the warmer water at the surface, closer to the air, has more dissolved oxygen than the colder "stagnant" water below. Different microorganisms thrive at different water depths, depending on their need for oxygen and nutrients. As the layers of water mix during fall and spring "turnover," organisms are stirred and dispersed. Water that is drawn from the reservoir during these biannual turbulent periods contains organisms different from the microorganisms drawn during "quieter" times of the year. Among these organisms may be algae and molds and even disease-causing agents such as bacteria and amoebas.

In industrialized countries, a water treatment plant works between the water supply and the tap to keep people healthy. Treatment plants filter and chlorinate water and are successful in removing most serious health threats, but they cannot remove everything or prevent growth after the water leaves the plant to make its way into our pipes. Microorganisms continue to flourish, particularly on the walls of water pipes and fixtures. When we shower, water from the shower head is broken up into droplets, some of them small enough to be inhaled. Most people can tolerate this because our lungs and immune systems protect us. For individuals weakened by immune disorders, smoking, or old age, however, water containing biological growth may cause disease.

Legionnaires' disease is a sometimes lethal form of pneumonia caused by a type of bacteria (*Legionella*) that grows best in warm water (see chapter 11). Though no cases I am aware of have been attributed to showers in homes, the disease has been caused by showers in hotels and hospitals. People have also acquired Legionnaires' disease from hot tubs after breathing bacteria aerosolized from the warm, frothy water.

Radon, a radioactive gas that causes lung cancer, is another threat to health. Where radon levels underground are high, well water contains the gas and carries the dissolved radon with it when it enters your home. When you shower, most of the radon gas bubbles out of the water and into the air, where you can breathe it in. Cities are required to test public water for radon, but homeowners are not. If you use well water, it's a good idea to purchase a test kit and have the water tested. It is estimated that for every ten thousand picocuries of radon radioactivity per liter in tap water, there will be about one picocurie in the air. (The EPA guideline for home exposure to radon in air is four picocuries per liter of air. See chapter 8 for further discussion of radon.)

RECOMMENDATIONS

THE TOILET

- If a toilet is loose or you smell sewer gas in your bathroom, even if the toilet seems secure, replace the wax ring.
- If condensation occurs on the outside of your toilet tank, put a tray under the tank to collect the water.

THE SINK

- If your sink leaks, have it repaired.
- Mold odors from a sink overflow can be eradicated with a mild bleach solution.

THE SHOWER AND TUB

- Keep the shower curtain inside the shower or be sure the shower doors are watertight. Do all you can to ensure that no water escapes the enclosure and gets onto the floor.

- Use tub splash guards with shower curtains.
- Replace shower curtains periodically.
- Keep shower doors clean. Remove slime from the tracks and clean those areas with a mild bleach solution.
- Cover windows in shower enclosures with waterproof curtains.
- If the escutcheon plate on a tub overflow is loose, the seal is leaking. Be sure the screws are tight and the rear seal is intact and seated properly.
- Drip awhile or dry yourself before stepping out of the shower or tub.
- Anything that becomes damp in the bathroom after showering should be allowed to dry. For example, don't let wet towels sit in clumps on the floor.
- Bathroom rugs should be cleaned regularly or replaced.
- If a rubber tub mat smells, soak it in diluted bleach.
- Operate a small fan to mix bathroom air after showering and to speed drying. The heat from a lamp will also help evaporate moisture. After showering, leave the lights on for a while with the bathroom door open.
- Instead of cornstarch, use bath powder made of talc, which is not a nutrient for microorganisms, sparingly.

THE ROOM

- Be sure your bathroom is adequately ventilated by a window, an exhaust fan, or both.
- To minimize mold growth, you can clean bathroom surfaces with a mild bleach solution. Clean off mold only while wearing an N95 NIOSH mask and ventilating the space to the exterior. A mild bleach solution will also kill mold on ceiling, walls, and grout.
- Repair any loose wall or floor tiles.
- Keep heat and air conditioning registers dust-free, particularly in a bathroom.

- If mildew tends to grow, avoid drying clothing in a bathroom.
- If you use well water, get a radon water test kit.
- If you are renovating and want to minimize the chances of mildew growth, insulate the bathroom walls and ceiling.

5

Living Rooms and Family Rooms

When we go to bed at night we lock our front doors, thinking we are keeping ourselves safe from any dangers that lurk outside. But what is inside our houses can also be threatening.

WOOD-BURNING FIREPLACES AND STOVES

A young mother was laying logs in the fireplace. Her infant, who had been asleep on the couch, began to awaken. The mother jumped up to keep the baby from rolling off, and in her haste she stubbed her toe badly against the coffee table. She was in such pain that she rushed to the emergency room, taking the baby with her and entirely forgetting about the open fireplace doors. In the middle of the night her husband was awakened by moaning coming from the bathroom. He found his wife sitting on the toilet, doubled over in pain from what he assumed was her recently injured toe.

As soon as the wife was back in bed, she heard a loud thud and looked down to see her husband unconscious on the floor. Luckily she suddenly realized that her nausea and her husband's collapse were the result of carbon monoxide poisoning. She threw open the bedroom window, ran to get the baby, and rushed back to her husband, who had already regained consciousness from the fresh air. Scantily dressed, the family fled into the freezing winter air.

I was asked to investigate why this happened. Warm air rises and cold air, which is denser, sinks. A chimney built in the middle of a house stays warm even when it's cold out because the chimney is surrounded by warm interior walls and warm air from the house rises through the flue, creating a draft.

This chimney, however, was built on the outside of the house. Unless there is a fire in the fireplace, an exterior chimney remains near the temperature of the outside air. In winter the colder air from outside sinks in such a chimney and enters the house. This is called downdrafting. The fire department determined that a defective boiler in the house was producing very high levels of carbon monoxide, a tasteless, odorless, but lethal gas. (How carbon monoxide forms is discussed later in this chapter.) The flue for the fireplace was next to the boiler flue in the same chimney. On that particular night, wind blew carbon monoxide gases from the boiler flue at the top of the chimney across to the adjacent fireplace flue, and they were carried down into the house through the fireplace doors, inadvertently left open. In the middle of the night the mother, father, and baby were within minutes of dying.

I have heard of similar cases occurring when the heating system flue was adjacent to the fireplace flue in an exterior chimney. For example, one older couple experienced intermittent headaches and nausea. They had the town health and fire departments test for carbon monoxide on numerous occasions, but none was ever detected because by the time the investigators arrived the wind had shifted. One investigator figured out what was happening and recommended that the couple keep their fireplace damper closed unless they were burning wood. That solved the problem.

It's a good idea in any case to keep the damper or doors closed when a fireplace is not in use. If you have a heating system with a flue in a chimney that also has a fireplace flue, be sure to maintain the system and have a technician check periodically for carbon monoxide levels in the combustion gases.

Carbon monoxide can also vent to the living space directly from the heating system flue itself, as one real estate agent learned. On a cold winter Sunday she was holding an open house in an older home. The house had three levels, with the kitchen and living room on the ground floor. On one side of the living room was a charmingly exposed interior brick chimney. Directly on the other side of the chimney was the mechanical room. The house was heated by a behemoth antique gravity hot-air heating system (see chapter 10) that had been converted from coal to gas.

Whenever she was in the house the broker wondered why the sellers kept the windows open. Perhaps they had something to hide, she thought, such as a musty odor. On her open house day she closed the windows to keep the house warmer. There was very little customer traffic, so she sat in the living room quietly reading. Suddenly she looked up from her book and the room swirled. She was so dizzy she had trouble making her way out of the house. She spent the rest of the open house sitting in the yard in the cold wind, trying to recover by taking deep breaths. Before she locked up she left a note warning the sellers, then she opened a few windows to leave the house as she had found it.

What had happened? The furnace's vent pipe connector was missing a large piece of metal at the top. This allowed combustion gases, which happened to contain a high level of carbon monoxide, to leak from the vent pipe into the mechanical room, and from there through the doorway into the living room. The real estate agent might as well have been sitting inside the chimney.

Downdrafting

Wood-burning stoves can be dangerous too. One couple told me about a near-death experience in their vacation cabin in the mountains. The cabin was on a steep hillside and was heated by a woodstove. The uninsulated metal chimney pipe exited the living room wall at the first floor, rose above the second floor at the outside of the cabin, and ended well below the peak of the roof.

Before the couple and their two young children went to sleep, the husband partially closed the stove's damper so the fire would last as long as possible into the night. The wind outside was sweeping down the hill, moving over the top of the chimney pipe, and hitting the peak of the roof. The cold outside air was forced down into the chimney, pushing the combustion products from the glowing embers back into the room through the combustion air hole at the front of the stove. Burning embers produce large amounts of carbon monoxide, and the cabin was filling with this deadly gas. The husband woke up nauseated and dizzy. Suspecting what was wrong, he opened all the windows to air out the house.

To remain in the house safely while the stove was burning wood, the family had to increase the draft going up the chimney. They kept the living room window on the uphill side open, and this did the trick. Why? Because the force of the wind coming down the hill and into the window increased the air pressure in the cabin, and this pushed air back up the chimney, carrying the combustion products with it. In other words, it reversed the downdraft.

In addition to posing health hazards, downdrafting can make it difficult to start a wood fire, particularly with an exterior chimney. In such cases the smoke can back up into the house. I once attended a formal housewarming party. The family had invited many friends to dinner in their new home. When they decided to use their fireplace for the first time, the noise of animated conversations was rising from groups all around the spacious living room. Smoke from the fireplace soon started to pour into the living room, where it rose and spread across the ceiling like a storm cloud. Even though the conversations began to be punctuated by coughs, no one complained about the cloud. Perhaps the guests didn't want to hurt their hosts' feelings.

Even without downdrafting, fireplaces and wood-burning stoves almost always create some smoke in homes. This can be irritating for children or adults who have asthma, so I recommend they avoid burning wood. Even if you have no allergies, if you are planning to install wood-burning devices and you live in a densely populated area, please consider the health of people with asthma who may be downwind.

I have another concern about wood. Some people may be allergic to molds or insects that grow in firewood. When wood is carried through the house or stored inside, allergens can enter the air or fall onto carpeting. If you can't resist the appeal of a working fireplace, your firewood should be moved and stored carefully.

Smoke Residues

Wood is composed mostly of cellulose (see chapter 1). When the cellulose burns, it first thermally decomposes (undergoes a chemical change because of heat), producing water vapor, wood alcohol vapor, and a complex mixture of other chemical vapors. What is left behind in the fireplace is charcoal (which eventually burns) and ash. The alcohol vapor, along with some of the other chemical vapors, burns in the flame. Smoke from the wood fire consists of droplets of water vapor and other unburned chemical vapors that have condensed when they hit cool air. Some of these chemicals, however, condense on the cooler chimney flue walls before they meet the outside air and form a tar-like coating called creosote. This coating continues to be exposed to the heat from the fire below, and it is baked into a combustible charcoal-like glaze. Much the same process happens when we bake an apple pie and the sugary filling oozes out and drips on the bottom of the oven, thermally decomposing into a black glaze. (Remember that cellulose and sugar both contain glucose.)

Creosote has a very strong odor, and where downdrafting occurs the entire house can smell of burned wood. Fireplace and woodstove flues that aren't kept clean fill up with creosote. One family I know had not been careful about having the chimney cleaned each year. One Christmas Day they threw a large bundle of wrapping paper from the presents into the fireplace all at once. The flames crackled, and suddenly a large *whoosh!* came from the chimney. The creosote lining the flue had caught fire, and flames filled the entire chimney. The house was in danger of burning to the ground, since the flames could have escaped the chimney, which was unlined and full of loose, deteriorated mortar. Even in lined chimneys the extreme heat from a creosote fire can cause a liner to expand, crack, and fail.

The family called the fire department, and the firemen quickly put out the fire. They also crunched a few of the presents as they walked in and out of the house in their heavy black boots. But better to lose a few presents than the entire house.

Creosote does have some useful applications. For years a solution of creosote and solvent was applied to wood as a preservative. This is the smell associated with old telephone poles. The odor of creosote can irritate some people, though. A builder I know was renovating his house for his fiancée. To preserve a decayed threshold leading from the living room to the exterior deck, he saturated the wood with an entire gallon of creosote solution. Whenever the woman entered the house, her lungs hurt. The builder removed the threshold as well as the concrete near the door and the creosote-soaked soil beneath. He replaced the concrete and threshold, but his fiancée continued to have trouble breathing in the house. Unfortunately, he had put so much creosote into the site that he couldn't remove it all. I recommended the couple install a subslab mitigation system similar to a radon system (described in chapter 8).

GAS FIREPLACES, CANDLES, AND SOOT

Gas fireplaces offer an easier way to create a romantic ambience than do wood-burning fireplaces. Instead of paying for wood, carrying it in, storing it in a corner, vacuuming up chips and sawdust, and cleaning out ashes, all you have to do is flick a switch. But gas fireplaces have drawbacks of their own.

Carbon monoxide is one by-product of a gas flame, the result of incomplete combustion. In complete combustion, one atom of carbon from fuel combines with two atoms of oxygen from air to produce carbon dioxide. In incomplete combustion, the carbon combines with one atom of oxygen, producing carbon monoxide. Because carbon monoxide can still combine with oxygen to form carbon dioxide, carbon monoxide burns in air. (To "burn" in air, a substance must be able to combine chemically with oxygen.)

Another problem caused by gas flames is soot. We expect kerosene and wood fires to create soot, but it's a surprise that gas flames can create soot as well. When gas burns normally in a stove, the flame is blue because adequate oxygen from air is premixed with the gas to complete combustion. When oxygen is inadequate, combustion is incomplete. Some carbon atoms combine with oxygen to create carbon dioxide while others combine with oxygen to create carbon monoxide. Still other carbon atoms do not combine with oxygen at all but combine with each other to produce soot—microscopic particles that become visible when present in large numbers. When these particles are heated in a flame, they become incandescent and give off the yellow light we associate with firelight. In gas logs in fireplaces, unlike stoves, the gas is not premixed with enough air before it burns, so that the fire will produce the yellow flame people want to see. Soot is the inevitable by-product. (Incandescent carbon particles also produce the yellow flame of wood and candles.)

One homeowner had his brother install a gas fireplace in an exterior living room chimney. There was not adequate draft, and carbon monoxide and soot leaked into the house. Even though the level of carbon monoxide was not high enough to make the people ill, looking at the soot deposits on the wall sickened them. They had to repaint their entire house.

Fireplaces aren't the only source of soot in a living room. Candles also can produce soot, some more than others. In recent years scented candles have become popular, and they can bother anyone sensitized to perfumes. Whether scented or not, candles burning in jars flicker more than candles burning freely in the air, because there are turbulent airflows around the jar rim. When the flame geometry is disturbed in this way, incomplete combustion occurs, producing even more soot.

In older homes, soot deposits are fairly uniform. In well-insulated newer homes, soot stains on exterior walls and on ceilings near exterior walls can look like stripes at the studs (the wood or metal wall supports the drywall is attached to) and black dots at nailheads. On an insulated exterior wall there is a temperature differential between the insulated bays and the studs. The studs are colder than the bays, and nailheads are even colder than the studs, for they penetrate deeper into the wall and conduct heat toward the outside of the building faster. The room air cools when it comes in contact with the nail-heads and with the plaster or drywall at the studs. This cooler air sinks, and a slight air turbulence occurs. Soot deposits increase as more air collides with surfaces, so that though soot sticks to the entire exposed surface, there are more deposits at the studs and nails.

Homeowners I know have repainted rooms more than once to cover soot stains. I heard about one contractor who had been sued by some of his buyers because the inside walls of some of the houses he had constructed turned black with soot. They blamed the soot on faulty installation of the heating system. As an experiment, he had an engineer burn a candle in a jar for sixty hours in a new home. So much soot was deposited that the entire interior had to be recarpeted and repainted. I know several people who have had to replace all their light-colored carpeting because of soot deposits from candles. In some rooms the stains were prominent at the edges where exterior walls met the carpet, probably because the colder air at the exterior wall sank, depositing more soot particles at that carpet edge.

In large buildings with basement parking garages, soot from automobile exhaust (particularly from cars with diesel engines) may enter hallways through airflows up the elevator shaft. If air from the common hallway gets into the apartment under the entry door, the carpeting there may develop a long, tongue-shaped soot stain. If you live in an apartment or condominium and your light carpet backs up to your unit's front door, you may have noticed this discolored "unwelcome mat."

Soot is made visible by its absence, as we notice when we move out of a

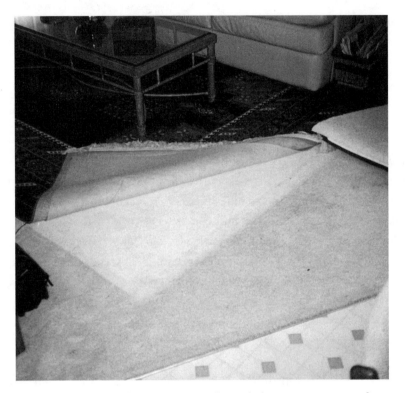

FIGURE 5.1. Carpet with soot staining. When a dark rug resting on top of a light carpet was folded back, it became clear that soot had discolored the exposed carpet. Invisible in air, soot is insidious; some people have found plastic utensils and containers inside kitchen cabinets and even refrigerators blackened by soot deposits.

house or apartment. When pictures are taken down, you can see the outline of the frame on the wall surface. The pictures protect the wall from the even layer of soot deposited elsewhere, so the area now uncovered looks lighter.

Soot is not just a cosmetic concern. People who have allergies or asthma may find that inhaling soot (along with other combustion products) is irritating. Soot also contains carcinogens (such as benzo[a]pyrene), so long-term exposure should be avoided. One final reason to forgo candles in jars is a recent finding that some of these candles produce unhealthy levels of lead in the air. Some manufacturers include a lead wire in the wick to make it stiffer so it will remain standing when not surrounded by wax. The heated lead becomes airborne and can be inhaled.

A HIDDEN BUZZ

In one home I inspected, I asked why many of the living room windows were taped shut. The seller told me that he was trying to keep bees out. I thought the bees were more likely entering through the fireplace, since I had seen what resembled a busy airport at the top of his tall chimney, with bees flying in and out. He asked if I thought a fire would "smoke them out." I recommended instead that he call a pest control operator (PCO) who specializes in bees to remove the nest.

Weeks later he called me to have his new home inspected, and I asked what had happened to the bees' nest in the residence he sold. He told quite a tale. The PCO wanted over $500 to do the job, so the fellow decided to smoke the bees out himself. The heat from the fire melted the wax in the nest, and half of the nest fell from the top of the chimney down into the fireplace. Dozens of bees entered the house, and the man was stung seven times before he escaped. (Luckily he wasn't allergic to bee stings!) But now the chimney was lined with wax and honey in addition to creosote and had to be cleaned.

In the living room of another home I inspected, I noticed a slight bubbling in the paint above a sliding door. The woman buying the house and both brokers watched as I crossed the room to have a closer look. When I pointed to it and accidentally touched the paint, a large section of the wall collapsed, leaving a big hole. The chunk that fell out consisted solely of paint, thinner than a piece of paper. There had been a bees' nest in the wall, and in expanding their nest the insects had removed all the plaster and paper from the drywall. Outside the sliding door was an obvious hole where bees had entered and exited. Luckily for me the nest was inactive.

This wasn't the case in another home. A woman noticed a stain on the wall of her family room. She rubbed her finger over it and discovered the sticky film was honey. She looked carefully over the wall and saw small drops of honey everywhere. She called a PCO, who found an active bees' nest within the wall cavities. He killed the bees and removed over fifty pounds of honey from the nest! In this case a small hole in the interior wall might have been deadly.

Each insect has its niche, and though it troubles me to see a honeybee nest destroyed, I do not recommend leaving beehives inside a home because someone may unknowingly have a life-threatening allergy to bee stings.

SUNKEN LIVING ROOM

I entered a very contentious scene when my client, a building manager, warned me to say "nothing to nobody" during the site visit. The disgruntled tenant was complaining of repeated bouts of mold growth on the lower six to twelve inches of the living room walls. The condominium owner (the landlord) had replaced the carpeting, then cleaned and repainted the living room. He had even growled to the management company about excessive moisture in the crawl space beneath the adjacent dining room, where dampness from the disconnected dryer vent hose was dripping from the steel beam.

Lint was in the crawl space and hostility was in the air. The "sunken" living room, slab on grade, had an outside wall with a glass sliding door and was about two feet below the level of the dining room and the rest of the apartment. The living room heat register was inappropriately high on the wall. I determined with an infrared thermometer that the lower two feet of the living room wall were significantly cooler than the wall above. I felt my legs chill below the knees and imagined myself standing in a bowl of stagnant cold air.

The bottom of the living room was in fact like a bowl of liquid, because it contained the denser, cold air. Once the lower two feet filled with the cooler air, the air spilled out over the two-foot-high wall between the living room and the dining room, where it mixed with warmer air. The temperature discontinuity therefore was occurring at the level of the adjacent dining room floor.

The moisture content of the air in the sunken living room was fairly uniform throughout, but the relative humidity was higher in the cooler portion of the room (as air temperature falls, the relative humidity rises). Consequently mildew grew on the living room walls. I explained that the tenant must not turn the thermostat down to 60°F every winter day before leaving for work and that he should move the furniture away from the cold walls so warmer room air could heat their surfaces. I suggested he do all he could to reduce moisture levels in the apartment by taking shorter hot showers and boiling less water on the stove. I also recommended that the landlord install an exhaust fan at the stove as well as a paddle fan in the living room to mix the stratified air and make the room air temperature more uniform. The building manager also needed to repair the disconnected dryer hose in the crawl space to prevent the dining room structure from decaying.

RESINOUS CEILINGS AND WALLS

In one case of mystery odor, a young couple purchased a derelict home and proceeded to renovate it while they were living there. They removed wallpaper, painted walls and trim, and refinished floors, but they were still plagued by an intermittent odor. This fleeting odor seemed strongest near a particular wall on cold days and at another end of the living room on other days. Some days there was no odor at all.

The odor was reminiscent of marijuana smoke. It occurred to me that all the walls and doors had newer finishes, but the ceilings had never been washed or painted. I borrowed a hair dryer and heated the living room ceiling. Within moments the couple agreed that the smell was suddenly present. Apparently the previous owners had used the drug so extensively that the ceilings were coated with resin from the smoke. On days when the steam heat operated, warm air would rise by convection above the living room radiator and heat the ceiling. The warm air would acquire the resin odor, move in an invisible air mass across the ceiling, and once cooled, sink at another wall. On other days the sun would heat parts of the room and create other convection pathways for the warmed air, causing the odor to appear elsewhere. The couple cleaned and painted the ceilings and the odor disappeared.

Tobacco use can cause similar problems. One family moved into a Victorian home with wainscoting in the living room and wood paneling in the family room. There was an omnipresent odor of pipe and cigar smoke in both rooms, yet no one in the family smoked. They had repainted the plaster walls and sanded the floors in the entire house before they moved in, but they had never cleaned the paneling or wainscoting. After they washed these wooden surfaces with a dilute solution of detergent and ammonia, the smell went away.

COUCH POTATO ASTHMA

One couple's teenage son found his asthma symptoms were worse whenever he was in their family room, where the TV and video games were. As a small child the boy used to lie on the couch and watch *Sesame Street*. As an elementary school student he played video games from the couch. As a teenager he would stay up late at night, lying on the couch and watching his favorite movies. The cushions were stuffed with down and offered a soft, comfortable retreat.

Unfortunately, as I discovered, the couch also offered an extremely high level of dust mite allergens. Dust mites love down (see chapter 3), and the skin scales and moisture from the boy's body supplied "mite feed." Whenever he moved around on the couch, compressing those cozy down cushions, clouds of sloughed-off skin scales and mite fecal pellets billowed out for him to breathe. He was allergic to mites, and the allergens exacerbated his asthma.

I recommended the family get rid of the couch with its down cushions and replace it with a leather or vinyl-covered one, or that they use a futon couch and encase the mattress in an allergen-control cover. Families with allergies or asthma should think carefully before purchasing furniture with down cushions, since these are promising reservoirs for microscopic life and, depending on one's lifestyle, can lead to what I call couch potato asthma.

In fact I believe a large portion of the increase in asthma can be attributed to our sedentary lifestyle. Years ago children and parents in this country spent much more time outdoors. Now family time is mostly dedicated to more passive pursuits such as playing video games, surfing the Internet, or watching TV. The longer we spend sitting on cushions or lying on mattresses and couches, the more favorable are the conditions for mite infestations.

GREENHOUSES AND HOT TUBS

Some homeowners add enclosures to their homes for hot tubs, pools, or plants. Such spaces can contribute more than an exotic flavor to a house. If you are thinking of adding a greenhouse, do all you can to control moisture levels. You will be introducing soil into the indoor spaces of your home, and whatever the soil contains may become airborne when disturbed. (Several cases of Legionnaires' disease have occurred after people had heavy indoor exposures to aerosolized dust from potting soil contaminated with *Legionella*.) Indoor hot tubs and pools are sources of moisture that can lead to bacteria, mold, and mite colonization, in addition to irritation from the chemicals used to disinfect the water. In one home a hot tub was the source of a powerful bacterial odor. I found the underside of the vinyl cover completely covered

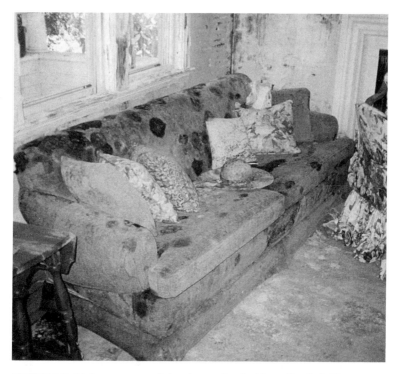

FIGURE 5.2. Living room couch in a home that had been flooded. This uninhabited home remained damp months after it was flooded by a broken pipe at the second floor, and mold grew on most surfaces. All the oval and round black stains on the couch were colonies of *Stachybotrys* mold, most of them probably started by a single mold spore.

with biological growth and mites. In another home with an indoor pool and a powerful mold odor, the pool cover was overgrown with a forest of *Aspergillus* mold, with mites foraging happily within. If you have a hot tub or pool with a cover, be sure both sides of the cover are dust-free and periodically disinfected.

Living rooms and family rooms are important in the private and public life of the household, so these spaces are well-trafficked by family members and guests alike. With this level of activity, whatever allergens and irritants are in the room will be stirred up and carried into other parts of the home by the airflows. Be sure to keep these rooms as dust-free, dry, and clean as possible.

FIREPLACES AND WOOD STOVES

- Be sure the damper, fireplace doors, or both are closed when the fireplace or wood-burning stove is not in use, particularly if you have an exterior chimney.
- If the boiler and fireplace flues are in the same exterior chimney, look into installing a damper that fits onto the top of the chimney flue.
- If allergens or mold affect you or anyone in your family, store the wood for your fireplace outside, but be sure the wood stays dry. Try to avoid burning moldy firewood.
- Keep a carbon monoxide detector in your house, particularly if you have a gas fireplace.
- Have chimneys and chimney vent piping cleaned regularly by a professional.
- Avoid creosote buildup in your chimney, and do not apply creosote-containing preservatives to surfaces in the interior of your home.

SOOT STAINS

- Don't burn candles (particularly those in jars) in well-insulated homes.

FURNITURE

- Use vinyl- or leather-covered furniture rather than upholstered furniture. Avoid down-filled furniture or cushions.
- If you have a sofa bed or futon in the living room, encase the mattress in an allergen-control cover.

MISCELLANEOUS

- To deter mildew growth, keep humidity at a minimum comfort level (under 40 percent in winter) and keep the living room or family room evenly heated.
- Periodically disinfect an indoor hot tub or pool cover and keep it as dust-free as possible.

6

Kitchens and Dining Areas

The kitchen and dining area are where we gather for our meals and our social lives and where we reconnect with other members of the household. As we obtain nourishment there, we need to be sure no unwelcome life forms do the same. We also want to be certain we prepare and cook foods safely.

STOVES
Cooking with Gas

A woman had experienced chronic headaches for all of the twenty years she had lived in her home. She loved to cook and spent a great deal of time in the kitchen or the adjacent dining area. She called me because she realized she always felt a little better when she spent extended time away from the house. I first sampled for gas sources in the basement with my TIF 8800 combustible gas detector. The clocklike ticking remained constant there, but as I ascended the stairs to the first floor the pulse began to increase. The closer I got to the kitchen stove, the faster it ticked. As I moved the detector along the back of the stove, it screeched with its characteristic siren sound. I soon found that gas was leaking from piping concealed in the wall behind and under the stove.

The gas company representative was fearful enough of an explosion that he cut off the gas to the kitchen and laundry. On the following day a plumber cut holes in the basement ceiling and walls and found three significant leaks in the gas piping joints. Once these were repaired the woman's headaches diminished. Her husband had never smelled the gas or had any headaches at all. The house had been built on fill, and the only thing that bothered him was that the house had sunk about six inches at one end. It's possible the settling had stressed the pipes and caused some of the leaks.

Even in the absence of leaks, you have to be careful with gas appliances. Newer gas stoves have a spark ignition coil to light the top burners and an electric glow plug to light the oven. If the automatic spark does not operate properly when a burner is turned on, gas will pour out around the stove. If ignition is then initiated (or if you try to light the stove with a match), the gas-air mixture can ignite and produce a large flame. Similar brief conflagrations in older, manually lit ovens have resulted in many a singed eyebrow! Accidents like these are also likely to occur with propane gas because it is denser than air and hangs around the stove. Utility-supplied gas is lighter (less dense) and thus rises and dilutes faster.

Older gas stoves lack automatic ignition mechanisms and instead have pilot lights that burn day and night. Occasionally pilot lights can cause disasters. My next door neighbors renovated their entire first-floor condominium. The walls were sparkling, and they had only the floors to refinish before the project was complete. They hired a refinishing company. The workers sanded the floors in the entire unit, vacuumed up all the sawdust, and applied a sealer coat of lacquer that contained a very volatile solvent. The fumes filled the apartment. Because they were denser than air, the fumes were concentrated in the space close to the floor. When the invisible cloud of solvent reached the oven pilot light, the vapor ignited. There was a *whoosh!* and the entire floor was ablaze. The fire flashed back to the open bucket of lacquer, setting it on fire too. The foolish floor sander tried to extinguish the flames by pouring the burning lacquer down the bathtub drain rather than covering the bucket with a plate or metal pot cover.

Fortunately no one was injured, and the burning floors self-extinguished once the volatiles had burned off. If there are solvents or any type of chemical fumes in a home, turn pilot lights off and keep the windows open. (A pilot doesn't produce much gas, but turning the gas to the appliance off altogether will stop gas leakage.) After the solvent vapors have cleared, it's safe to light the pilots or turn on the gas.

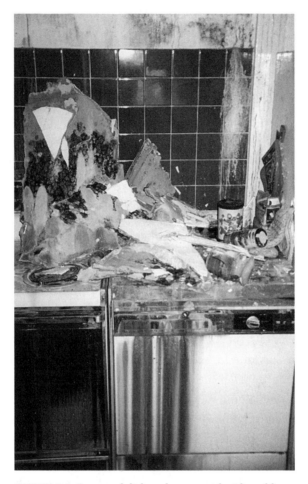

FIGURE 6.1. Stove and dishwasher covered with moldy drywall. A couple renovated their house and then went on an extended vacation. A pipe leaked the entire time they were away, and water soaked into the ceiling above their new kitchen. The weight of the wet drywall caused the ceiling to collapse onto the dishwasher and stove. *Stachybotrys* mold had been flourishing on the back of the drywall. The rust stains on the dishwasher show that the water had leaked for many weeks.

Carbon Monoxide

Pilot lights on older stoves can produce significant amounts of carbon monoxide. In addition, if there are minor gas leaks in the kitchen piping, the hot pilot light thermally decomposes the gas-air mixture in the room air to produce carbon monoxide and emits a characteristic odor that I often associate with kitchens in older homes. (When homes are painted with oil paint, the hot gas flame of a pilot light or burner thermally decomposes the solvent vapor and can produce a pungent, irritating odor.) Whether you have an older or a newer gas stove, a poorly adjusted flame on a burner or in the oven can produce significant amounts of carbon monoxide. Gas ovens should be tested periodically for carbon monoxide and should never be used to heat a home.

One woman who was renting her apartment called me because a peculiar odor in her unit was making her nauseated. She had been able to live there for only one week; in fact on the day she moved in she called the gas company and the fire department because she was so worried. They found no problem and questioned her mental health. The building owner recommended she install a portable air filter.

I could detect the odor of combustion gases as soon as I entered her apartment, so I went out to my car to get my Bacharach Monoxor II carbon monoxide detector. At 800 parts per million (ppm), carbon monoxide can cause loss of consciousness and death within hours; the maximum allowable short-term exposure in a home is 9 ppm. Fortunately the level of carbon monoxide was low, 5 ppm, but it was enough to be of concern. (The level in the uninhabited apartment should have been zero!) The gas pipe that supplied her cooking stove was in the basement. The pipe had not been properly threaded into a fitting, and a large amount of gas was leaking from the joint and rising up into her kitchen. I told her to call the gas company and request an immediate service call. A technician came and was so alarmed that he turned off the gas supply in the basement.

Self-cleaning electric ovens produce carbon monoxide when on the automatic cleaning cycle. This is caused by thermal decomposition of the food in the oven as it is heated and burned off by the red-hot coils. If you have ever experienced nausea or headache in a closed kitchen during the oven's self-cleaning cycle, carbon monoxide may have contributed. To whatever extent possible, keep the kitchen doors and windows open and the exhaust fan on when your oven is self-cleaning.

Some people love the taste of grilled foods, but a charcoal barbecue should never be used in the kitchen or anywhere indoors. Not only does this present a fire hazard, but glowing or burning charcoal—which is mostly carbon—produces vast amounts of carbon monoxide. Carbon monoxide is formed when oxygen and carbon combine in the presence of heat. We light charcoal by pouring lighter fluid (kerosene) on it and then lighting the fluid. As the fluid heats it turns to vapor, which then burns with a flame. The charcoal then heats up in the flame, and the oxygen in the air at the charcoal's surface combines with the carbon to produce carbon monoxide. It is the carbon monoxide gas that burns with a flame after the lighter fluid has been consumed.

(Only burning vapor or burning gas produces a flame. A candle illustrates this process. The wick is covered with wax, which we light with a match. The match flame melts the wax on the wick and heats the liquid wax, creating a vapor, which then ignites into a flame. The heat from the flame melts the wax in the candle, which the wick then soaks up. The heat turns that wax into vapor, and on it goes.)

Blackened Food

It's easy to overheat foods. Occasionally burned foods can create air quality problems. My family discovered this when our teenage son, proud of his cooking skills, offered to prepare a spaghetti dinner using his special sauce recipe. Unlike most of us in the family, he likes hot, spicy food. He began by heating oil in a large cast-iron frying pan. He added fresh chopped jalapeño peppers. Next he cut up an onion and threw it into the hot oil. Grease spattered. Shortly afterward I heard a loud commotion in the kitchen. My son was coughing, and his face was flushed. He had overheated the frying pan and found the clouds from the cooking vegetables so irritating that before I came he shoveled the mixture into the disposer. As soon as I entered the kitchen I also started coughing, even though the cooking had stopped. My wife rushed in and immediately felt a burning sensation in her lungs. We turned off the stove and threw open all the windows to air out the room.

I asked my son what had happened. He was not quite forthcoming, because he wanted to keep the peppers a "secret." He said he had burned the onions, which then filled the room with smoke. I took bits of the leftover onion skin from the cutting table and looked at them under the microscope. I found several types of mold growing, including *Stachybotrys,* the mold that produces trichothecene mycotoxin. I had no idea whether the mycotoxin could have caused our distress, but since we were all affected I was so concerned that, even though it was evening, I called a mycologist (a specialist on molds).

Imagine my embarrassment when my son finally admitted there had been jalapeño peppers in the pan. These peppers contain a very irritating chemical, capsaicin, as you may have discovered if you have ever chomped on one. Capsaicin is an ingredient in some pepper sprays that even police use for personal protection. When the peppers were fried, some of the irritant dissolved into the oil. As the moisture in the onions began to boil, the oil spattered into small droplets and dispersed into the air.

The oil aerosolized because when water boils it changes from liquid to vapor. When this happens in hot oil, the process is like an explosion. One teaspoon of liquid water becomes a thousand teaspoons of water vapor because vapor takes up more space than liquid (the molecules in vapor are farther apart). The volume change creates bubbles of water vapor in the oil that burst, spattering the oil and making the sizzling sound we associate with frying.

Even before food is added to the pan, any kind of overheated fat can thermally decompose and produce noxious smoke that contains acrolein, another very pungent, irritating chemical. Worse, the smoke can erupt into flames. Never pour water on such a fire; the ensuing spattering only makes the flames worse. The simplest way to extinguish a grease or oil fire instantly is to remove the source of oxygen by covering the pan.

Exhaust Systems

Cooking smoke consists of water vapor and droplets of water and grease. If the grease droplets are small enough, they remain suspended in the air and are carried by convection currents to walls, ceilings, windows, and shelves. After the droplets collide with surfaces, they coalesce into a sticky film. On vertical surfaces the yellowish film may not be apparent, though it makes blue walls look green. On horizontal surfaces like the top of the refrigerator or window rails, the film is very visible because house dust settles into it.

Grease droplets can also be deposited in rooms adjacent to the kitchen. One dining room had a ceiling light fixture with five small lightbulbs. A foot above the fixture were five yellow stains that mirrored the arrangement of the lamps. When the fixture was on, warm air rose from each bulb by convection, carrying droplets of grease that stuck to the ceiling directly above the bulbs.

In another home the new owners were plagued by the odor of curry every time the heating system came on. The former owners had loved to fry foods with curry powder. When the heat was on the warm radiators created a current of air, drawing kitchen air across the outside of the cast iron radiator pipes. Droplets of grease containing fragrant curry seasonings were carried along with the air, and they collided with the radiator pipes and stuck. Whenever the radiators became warm they would reintroduce the aroma into the house air. The new owners washed the radiators with detergent and TSP (trisodium phosphate, a cleaning agent), and the curry smell went away.

Since the smoke and steam produced in cooking can create IAQ problems, I always recommend stove exhaust fans. Be sure to get one that has a squirrel-cage blower and not a propeller fan (propeller fans do not have adequate capacity). It's also extremely important that exhaust fans be vented to the outside. Otherwise the cooking fumes are blown right back into the interior air. To find out whether your exhaust is working properly, check the exterior vent when the fan is on to be sure the damper opens. Sometimes these dampers stick shut or become blocked with the nests of birds or bees.

PANTRY PESTS

In your pantry may lurk some unwelcome life forms such as mice, cockroaches, ants, flour moths, and storage beetles and mites. Body parts and fecal material from any of these creatures can be present in infested foods. It is always possible that someone will develop an allergic sensitivity after eating contaminated foods over a long period.

Flour moths are small (about 0.4 inch or 10 mm) grayish brown slow-flying insects whose larvae live on grains, such as flour and cereal, and in baked products such as cookies, crackers, pretzels, and other snack foods, including nuts and raisins. It's easy to acquire a flour moth infestation. If you borrow a box of crackers from an infected house or buy grains or dry pet food from a moth-ridden supermarket, it's likely you will import eggs and larvae into your home. The eggs hatch into larvae with big appetites. When mature, the larvae find hidden places to pupate into moths.

I first became aware of flour moths when I saw them flying in large circles around my pantry. I didn't do anything about them for some time. Then one day I walked into the pantry to see a jungle of writhing larvae dangling from threads stuck to the ceiling. It was like a scene from an Alfred Hitchcock horror film.

I opened a box of crackers and it was full of crumbs stuck together by fine threads. Inside a bag of flour, the white powder was writhing and full of fine filaments of larvae thread. I ended up throwing out everything but the canned goods, and these I washed, because larvae were pupating behind the paper labels. The larvae were even in cracks between the shelves and the wall, so I realized I could never kill them all. I abandoned the pantry and kept the door shut for about two weeks. I checked every day and was able to kill the newly hatched moths because they flew so slowly. Finally, after a few weeks, new moths stopped appearing so I knew the nightmare had come to an end. If you have a moth infestation, don't use pesticides. Be patient and take a more cautious approach.

REFRIGERATORS
Drips

Because stoves contain fire, people approach them with caution and respect. The same cannot be said of refrigerators. One client was awakened in the middle of the night by an enormous crash. He turned on the lights and wandered around trying to locate the source. When he got to the kitchen he realized in his sleepy stupor that something was missing. Where the refrigerator had been there was now a gaping hole in the floor. He looked down and there was his refrigerator, lying in the basement. The rotted floor under it had finally failed—the victim of years of leakage from the icemaker's water line.

In another home I inspected, water from a refrigerator leaked between the flooring and the subfloor. Moisture ran along the plywood, causing decay in the kitchen and dining room. Both floors had to be replaced. Leakage from these lines can be very subtle. Occasionally I have found oak flooring buckled in front of the refrigerator, one of the few obvious signs of this problem. Obscure water seepage can be detected with a Tramex moisture meter. If you don't have a meter, you should check with a flashlight under the refrigerator and at the icemaker's water line for signs of leaks.

Even refrigerators that don't have water lines can harbor mold. Some frost-free refrigerators have a drip tray at the bottom that collects water. The water drains from the freezer section during the defrost cycle or from the bottom of the refrigerator section when liquids are spilled inside. The drip tray in most homes also collects a considerable amount of house dust and bits of food.

At one point I coughed intermittently in my own kitchen. I never understood why until one day I realized that my coughing always began shortly after the refrigerator compressor started. I removed the grille at the bottom and looked inside. Somehow a small onion had bounced along the floor and ended up in the drip tray. The onion was fuzzy with a thick beard of blue-green *Penicillium* mold. Every time a refrigerator compressor turns on, room air is drawn over the coils that dissipate the heat from inside the refrigerator. By design, this air is used to evaporate water that accumulates in the drip tray. When the compressor in my refrigerator turned on, air blew over the moldy onion and spewed spores into the room.

Ever since then I've been careful to keep the drip tray clean, and people with asthma or allergies should do the same. In addition, you can add a few tablespoons of salt to the drip tray (as long as it's a plastic tray, since salt corrodes metal) to help minimize the growth of mold and bacteria.

The refrigerator coil is another item to keep clean. If you have pet allergies and a previous resident had a pet, it's especially important to clean the coil. The dust that accumulates on it, and around the refrigerator itself, can remain allergenic for years.

Mold Munchies

Refrigerator doors can be a source of mold and odor if the gasket seal is poor or broken and food falls into the spaces. In damp weather moisture condenses on the cooler gasket surface: combine the nutrients and moisture, and voilà! Mold. Try to keep the gaskets clean, and if they are damaged, replace them. So much moisture had condensed on one refrigerator gasket that it was covered with mold, and mites were happily foraging on the crop.

It's common sense to keep the inside of your refrigerator free of moldy foods, but many foods like cheeses include molds intended to be eaten. The

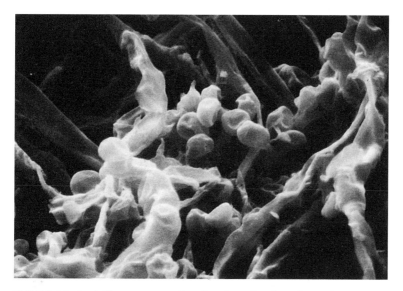

FIGURE 6.2. *Penicillium* spores and hyphae from the skin of Brie cheese. This skin is not cheese at all but is made up of *Penicillium* spores and hyphae. The *Penicillium* spores, which are normally oval, and the hyphae, which are normally tubelike, look puckered because they were desiccated during the vacuum process required to prepare the sample for the scanning electron micrograph. (2,500× SEM)

white skin on Brie and Camembert, for example, consists primarily of *Penicillium* hyphae (and spores). Blue cheese is made by fermenting milk curd with *Penicillium roqueforti,* which sometimes also contains *P. crustosum* (another species of *Penicillium* that produces a nervous system toxin that can kill animals when they eat contaminated grain). People who are allergic to mold may react to such fermented foods. In fact, people with food allergies can be so sensitized that just being in the same room with someone eating a food such as peanuts or walnuts can make them ill. Particulates from the nuts become airborne and the sufferer inhales them.

Moldy foods (fruit, bread, or discolored cheese) should not be eaten by people with allergies. Keep in mind that moldy food, even when being thrown out, can emit irritating spores, either on the way to the garbage or while in the garbage can. Carefully place very moldy food in a bag, seal the bag, then remove it from the kitchen.

Whether you have food allergies or not, always remember to leave the refrigerator door open if you unplug the appliance. Whatever food is left inside (including food that is spattered on the walls, not all of which you can readily see) will be fodder for mold and bacteria.

Some people get headaches or feel sick when they smell rotting foods, so garbage should not be kept indoors for long (for this discussion, garbage includes compost). Disposers can also smell, particularly in hot weather, because they retain foods that are being decomposed by bacteria or mold. When you use your disposer, be sure all the food is ground up. In addition, you can pour a mild bleach solution into the disposer to eliminate bad smells. After adding bleach, be sure to run water through the disposer for a few moments before turning it on. Otherwise bleach might splash out.

OTHER SMELLY SPOTS
Leaky Sinks and Putrid Wipes

If your kitchen sink has a long-standing leak—whether around the faucets, behind the backsplash, or in the pipes underneath—then the counter and the cabinet can rot and smell. Nearly every sink sprayer I have seen leaked from the fitting in the spray handle. When this happens the water runs down the hose and drips into the base cabinet. It's a good idea to move stored goods periodically to check for leaks.

You should use as little water as possible throughout your kitchen, even when wiping counters, so that moisture does not seep into the countertop (most often particle board made from sawdust) and cause swelling and cracking. These spaces can become catchalls for food bits, and when moisture is added they become a pest and pestilence heaven. Sponges help contain water, but because of their open-celled structure they soak up food and become sources of bacteria and odor. One type of bacteria that grows in sponges is *Pseudomonas;* some species cause illnesses in people and animals.

In a number of my odor investigations a dirty sponge has turned out to be the culprit. The conference room in a law office had been abandoned because whenever the attorneys met there they experienced headaches and nausea. This is not a lawyer joke—there actually was a problem. The moment I entered the room I could smell the unpleasant odor. I took air samples and checked surfaces, but I couldn't find the source. The last item to check was the enormous oval mahogany conference table. The only thing on the table was

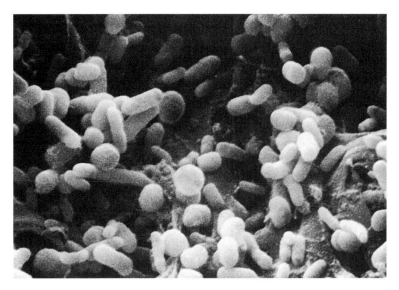

FIGURE 6.3. Bacteria on a sponge. Someone used this sponge to wipe up milk and did not rinse it afterward. Bacteria grew in the nutrients, and the sponge began to smell sour. The photomicrograph depicts different types of bacteria: rods, which are elongated, and cocci, which are round. The longer rods that seem pinched in the center are in the process of dividing. (10,000× SEM)

the Yellow Pages. I picked up the phone book and sniffed the top. There was no odor at all. But the side that had been against the tabletop had a powerful odor of dirty sponge. I had one of the lawyers repeat this test. She sniffed the top of the phone book and smelled nothing. When she smelled the bottom, she blurted out, "That's it!"

The lawyers often met over lunch, and afterward someone always wiped the table with a sponge from the kitchenette in the corner. The guilty sponge must have been full of bacteria, which were then spread over the table in a slimy, odoriferous film. When the film dried the smell remained. A chemical called butyric acid—a by-product of bacterial growth—causes this type of odor. (In the stomach, enzymes digesting fats convert them to butyric acid; when we throw up, it smells like a dirty sponge.)

Since butyric acid is an acid, it can be neutralized by a base (acid and base, when mixed in the right proportions, may produce a substance in water that is neither acidic nor basic). I sprayed and wiped the table three times with a window cleaner containing ammonia (a base), and the odor was gone. I called the next day at lunch hour, and once again the conference room was in use. I reminded them to wipe the table with a clean sponge! (Soaking a smelly sponge in diluted ammonia will eliminate odor and kill bacteria.)

Some people find the odor of ammonia objectionable; a little baking soda in water will also neutralize butyric acid. If you use a baking soda solution, be sure to rinse and dry the surface thoroughly afterward. Ammonia is a gas dissolved in water, so when the water evaporates the ammonia goes with it. Baking soda is a solid, and when the water in a baking soda solution evaporates, crystals of soda remain behind.

My experience with the smelly conference table helped me invent a simple test that many of my clients have used to find odor sources, particularly if a whole space is affected. If you suspect a surface is generating an odor of some kind, try the "foil test" described in the recommendations at the end of chapter 2.

Dishwashers

My new dishwasher could have burned my house down. When the appliance was first installed, it had a strong plastic odor that I found irritating. The odor got worse when the dishwasher was running, particularly on the dry cycle. I assumed the plastic was off-gassing and that the odor would go away with time, but it remained for months. One day in the middle of the dry cycle, the dishwasher ground to a halt. The repair person took off the front panel and unscrewed the electric junction box cover. He discovered that the wires had not been secured properly by the wire nuts. The poor electrical connection led to arcing and heating. The plastic wire nuts were melted almost beyond recognition. If you detect a strange odor coming from your dishwasher, trust your instincts and call for a repair.

When dishwashers are in good working order, water in the wash cycle is splashing around inside the machine. The interior is open to the kitchen through an air vent in the door. The splashing creates very small droplets that can exit the machine with airflows. The droplets contain small amounts of detergent that can be irritating to those who are sensitized. If my clients say this bothers them, I suggest they stay out of the kitchen when the dishwasher is on or try another detergent (but use only no-suds detergent specifically formulated for dishwashers).

I also recommend that in the summertime people rinse the plates thoroughly before placing them in the dishwasher or that they use the "rinse and hold" cycle if the dishes will be sitting in the machine for a while before the complete wash cycle. Don't let water sit in the bottom of the dishwasher: bacteria will grow in the food bits, and the dishwasher will start to smell rotten.

Heaters

A couple thinking of purchasing a luxury unit in a complex on a wharf jutting out into a harbor asked me to inspect the property. Because the building was literally "on the water" there was no basement, only a crawl space. While inspecting the exterior I noted that several screened covers to the crawl space vents were missing. Inside the unit, I noticed that someone had placed plastic from a garbage bag between the heat register and the floor to prevent air from blowing out.

The register was in the kitchen floor right next to the sink—a poor location for such a heat supply. One could easily imagine all sorts of food scraps falling into it. Curious about the condition of the duct, I removed the register and then the plastic beneath it. I noticed the fiberglass insulation inside the duct was chewed, and then I realized what was happening. The plastic ducts for the unit all ran through the inaccessible crawl space; rodents had access from the wharf because of the missing vent screens, and they had chewed through the ducts, attracted by the food that fell into the registers. Can you imagine peeling carrots at the sink and looking down to see an unwelcome guest nibbling on the scraps? I recommended that my buyers replace all the flexible plastic ducts in the crawl space with metal ones and that they be careful not to drop food. In addition, they could move the register away from the sink (and ask the condo association to replace the crawl space vent screens).

My wife had her own problem with a heat register near the sink and refrigerator. When our children were toddlers, their toys were often scattered across the kitchen floor. One day she took an opened half gallon of milk from the refrigerator. On her way to the sink she tripped over a toy and dropped the milk carton, which fell onto the heat register at her feet, emptying much of its contents into the duct below—a pretty unusual way to heat milk! I made certain to eliminate all the milk, since any residue could ferment and be a constant source of sour odor as warm air entered the kitchen.

In homes with forced hot-water heat rather than hot-air heating, a heater may be installed in the kickspace under the kitchen cabinets because there is no room for baseboard convectors or radiators. A blower forces air across coils containing hot water and then out of the kickspace. Food often gets into the space and can never be cleaned out unless there is an access panel at the bottom of the cabinet. In one home I sampled the air coming out of the blower and found large numbers of mold spores. In another house I found a layer of mouse droppings almost an eighth of an inch thick around the blower.

Another problem with kickspace heaters is the source of makeup air. When the blower is operating it usually doesn't take in air from the kitchen; it draws air from beneath the cabinets or wherever else it can get it. Very often this air comes from a moldy basement through holes around the pipes rising through the cabinets.

If you have a kickspace heater in your kitchen, make sure there is an access to the blower for cleaning and that there is a way for air from the kitchen to flow into the kickspace. You may need to seal around the pipes from the basement.

DINING AREAS

One family installed a kickspace heater in their dining room addition. This was unusual, but their plumber told them it would be less expensive to have a single blower under the stairway leading to the dining room than to install baseboard convectors on the walls of the room. There was no opening in the habitable area for makeup air for the heater, so the blower drew in the air it needed from the basement and the moldy crawl space under the addition. The couple's son experienced asthma symptoms soon after the addition was completed, and it turned out he was allergic to molds, which of course were being circulated by the heater. (He was so allergic to the air in the moldy basement that he ventured down only with a face mask!)

Some people have separate dining rooms and some people have eat-in kitchens or a combined kitchen, dining area, and family room. Whatever the configuration in your home, if you have a rug under your table, take great care to vacuum up food that drops on the floor. I never recommend carpeting or rugs in a kitchen, where food and moisture support biological growth. I also caution people against using jar candles, even though they contribute a romantic ambience to dining. (See chapter 5 for a discussion of the hazards of candle fragrance and soot.)

RECOMMENDATIONS

COOKING FOOD

- If you have a gas stove, be sure there are no leaks.
- Always be sure the ignition is on when you turn on a gas burner.
- On older gas stoves, be sure all the pilot lights are lit.
- Never use flammable liquids around pilot lights.
- Once in a while, put a carbon monoxide detector in the kitchen when you are baking with a gas oven.
- Keep the windows open when operating any stove on the self-clean cycle.
- Never use a charcoal grill inside the house.
- Have an adequate vented exhaust fan (with a squirrel-cage blower) over the oven and stove and use it.
- To minimize cooking odors in the kitchen and the rest of the house, keep the walls and other surfaces free of grease.

PANTRIES

- Keep grain foods tightly sealed in plastic.
- If you see a flour moth in a supermarket, don't buy grain foods there.

REFRIGERATORS

- If your refrigerator supplies ice or cold water, check the water line for leaks by looking behind with a bright light.
- If the refrigerator has a plastic drip tray, keep two tablespoons of salt

in it. Keep any drip tray clean and the area around and below the refrigerator free of dust.

- Replace broken gaskets.
- Keep the refrigerator coils dust-free. Vacuum periodically with a suitable attachment.

ODORS

- Get rid of your garbage quickly.
- A dilute bleach solution will remove smells from a disposer.
- A mild ammonia solution will remove a rotten sponge smell from a surface.
- Smelly sponges can be soaked in an ammonia solution to remove the odor. But remember, *never* mix bleach with ammonia: this creates chloramine, a toxic gas.

HEATERS

- The area around kickspace heaters should have an access panel and should be kept clean, and the makeup air should come from the habitable space rather than from the basement or crawl space.

MISCELLANEOUS

- If you use rugs and carpets in areas where food is prepared and served, keep them clean and dry.

7

Laundries

Having a washer and dryer in the house is a great convenience, but if we aren't careful the machines can make the air in our homes dirty even as they're making our clothes clean.

LAUNDRY DISEASE

Referred by her concerned pulmonologist, a retired woman called me because she was facing a third bout of lung surgery for aspergillosis, a relatively untreatable disease in which *Aspergillus* mold actually grows in the lungs. The first floor of her home was open to the basement, where she spent several hours each day working on hobbies. The woman cleaned the basement using a shop vacuum; these machines are notoriously leaky and spread many particulates into the air. She also did her laundry in the basement. Behind the washer and dryer I saw a large piece of plywood with dark stains at the bottom. The water supply to the washing machine had a slow leak, and the water had been soaking into the plywood. The dryer hose was partially disconnected, so air from the dryer blew against the plywood.

I took samples of the dust from the stained plywood, and I could see with a microscope that it consisted almost entirely of *Aspergillus* mold. There was even *Aspergillus* in the dust on top of the asbestos insulation on the steam pipe. The leaking exhaust from the dryer blew the mold spores into the air, and some went into the woman's lungs with every breath. Once the problem was solved, she began to recover. Her pulmonologist prescribed steroids and

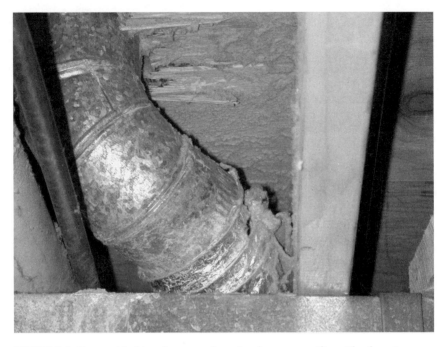

FIGURE 7.1. Torn and leaking dryer vent hose in a basement ceiling. The dryer is on the first floor, directly above. The flexible aluminum dryer hose beneath the dryer is torn and loose where it connects to the metal elbow. Lint is accumulating on the joist and plywood subfloor. In this home, the inhabitants did not do much laundry. In other homes, this condition can lead to moisture condensation in the ducts and the growth and release of mold spores.

canceled the surgery. She felt so much better she took a cruise around the world.

On another home inspection I discovered a large mushroom growing on the main beam in the house. There was significant discoloration and decay of the wood. I traced the discoloration back to one of the floor joists that was directly beneath the washing machine. When I looked behind the washer with a mirror and flashlight, I could see a glistening drop of water hanging from one of the black supply hoses. The threaded fitting at the end of the hose was completely rusted and had been leaking for years.

One homeowner with allergies had symptoms whenever he was near the laundry area, in a closet off a carpeted second-floor hallway. The carpet extended beneath the washer and dryer. I took Burkard air samples in the house and found that the air in the hallway contained many more mold spores than the air in the rest of the house. The washing machine had been leaking unnoticed, and mold was growing in the damp carpet. The man's symptoms subsided after he fixed the washing machine, replaced the hall carpet, and had a vinyl floor laid in the laundry area.

In the garage on a purchase inspection, I found a washing machine hose with a bulge the size of a grapefruit, just about to burst. I don't test appliances on home inspections, but during another inspection a buyer operated the washing machine and forgot to turn off the plumbing valves when he left the property. Over the weekend the washing machine hose burst in the unoccupied unit, flooding and destroying it. This is why I recommend using stainless steel-covered laundry hoses and turning off the water supply when a washer isn't in use. This is particularly important when the machine is not in the basement. When laundry appliances are installed on the first or second floor in closets or in kitchen extensions, a floor drain piped into a basement sink should be added, if possible, to handle any leaks. Occasionally these drains are piped into the house drain system, but the drain must have a trap to prevent sewer gas from entering the house. A trap can function only if there is water in it, however. If you have a drain of this kind, pour a cup of water into it about once a month to keep odors out of the house.

Detergent Blues

Detergents and fabric softeners contain chemicals (including fragrances) that some people find irritating to breathe. When the washing machine is operating, very small amounts of these chemicals enter the air. As the water is agitated, bubbles float to the surface because they are less dense than the liquid. When a bubble reaches the surface it pops through, and the thin water film at the top of the bubble (the cap) breaks. The surface of the water beneath the cap springs up and ejects a droplet of soapy liquid.

Some of these droplets enter the air even though the washer lid is closed. When the machine refills after emptying, the water displaces air that contains droplets, and even more irritants are emitted into the room. Some of these droplets are so small they become suspended in air, where they and the laundry chemicals they contain may be inhaled. For this reason, people with allergies and asthma should avoid using perfumed detergents and liquid fabric softeners.

One of my clients had a laundry in a hallway outside her child's bedroom. The boy had asthma, and his symptoms seemed to increase on washday. I recommended the family do the laundry when the son was in school, because the droplets released persist for only a short time. They quickly settle out of the air or leak out of the house with airflow, which can be increased by opening a window.

DIRTY AND CLEAN

How you handle the clothing before and after it's washed can also affect indoor air quality. Most people put dirty clothes in a hamper; some let them accumulate on the basement floor if the laundry area is on that level. Either way, if some of the dirty clothing is damp, within hours bacteria may start to grow on skin scales or on the cellulose fibers in cotton, particularly in warm weather. If the clothes are left long enough, mold may begin to flourish. In a basement of one unusual property I was inspecting, the lighting was poor, but I could see large piles of clothing on the floor. The scene reminded me of a mountain range except that the air wasn't fresh. When I looked more closely I could see that the soiled clothing had been there for months, and mushrooms were growing on some of the piles. I wouldn't suggest wearing it again!

Some homes have laundry chutes, and the clothing sometimes ends up on the basement floor waiting to be washed. Don't leave the piles there too long, particularly if the basement is damp. As a home inspector, I also have a safety concern about laundry chutes. They should have secured doors to prevent a child from falling in. I heard about one family in which an older child dropped the youngest down the chute as a joke. Luckily he landed on a pile of clothing—the very pile I just recommended you not accumulate.

After clothing is washed, it's not a good idea to leave it wet for too many hours because, again, bacteria may start to grow. If this happens you can rewash the clothes with some ammonia in the water, but never mix ammonia with bleach.

Occasionally washing machines themselves have a strong sour odor. Although the tub may look clean, the space around the agitator shaft can fill with wet lint that can be degraded by bacteria or mold. To clean this area you have to remove the agitator and clean the inside of the shaft as well as the outside. If the shaft in your washing machine has a basket at the top to capture lint, this too should be cleaned out periodically.

DRYING CLOTHES

During the energy crisis in the 1970s, many experts recommended venting dryers directly into living spaces to add moisture. This suggestion was based on the theory that moist air feels warmer, so people could be comfortable at lower house temperatures. (For example, room air at 70°F feels like 65°F at 20 percent relative humidity but like 71°F at 80 percent.) Some homeowners also thought they would be wasting heat if they vented a dryer to the outside. A dryer that is vented into the house will indeed add heat and moisture, but it will also add lint. To combat this problem, some people added a "lint trap"— a plastic device half filled with water that looks like a barrel with holes in it. A lint trap does not contain all the lint, and what lint it does catch becomes damp and can then support mold growth.

Dryers should always be vented directly to the outside or they will spew excess moisture and lint—coated with laundry chemicals—into the house. In addition, gas dryers may also exhaust carbon monoxide. Some people think venting the dryer into the garage is sufficient. On one of my first "sick house" inspections, I looked at a home for a fellow who was highly allergic to mold. When I arrived he greeted me and led me into his kitchen, where he was preparing his lunch. On the table was a large cardboard box full of dozens of bottles of vitamins, vegetable extracts, and other health remedies.

He and I walked around the home, and when I came to the laundry I noticed the dryer hose was venting directly into the garage. I looked in the garage and was met with an amazing sight. Water was dripping down the glass windows of the overhead door, because each load of laundry evaporates up to twenty pounds of water, the difference between the weight of a wet load and a dry load. Lint was stuck to every surface, and mold was growing on all the walls. The man was exposed to mold spores every time he went into the garage.

One afternoon I was inspecting a multifamily house and was in the basement while the tenant was doing his laundry. The dryer exhaust was venting directly into the basement, and there was a layer of lint on everything. I heard

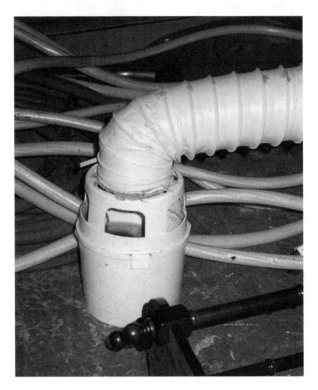

FIGURE 7.2. Dryer lint trap venting into a crawl space. Water condensed in the trap, and lint that collected in the water became moldy. (The contaminated water can be seen through one of the rectangular openings in the trap.) Air from the dryer blew mold spores into the crawl space, and the spores were drawn back into the house by leaky furnace return air ducts. The homeowner was very allergic to mold.

a commotion from the other side of the basement and saw flames coming out of the dryer. The terrified man turned off the dryer and managed to extinguish the fire. Lint had built up at the air intake, close to the gas flame, and ignited!

The moisture and lint entering the house from an incorrectly vented dryer can cause all sorts of problems. A fellow home inspector sent me an article from a newspaper in Virginia describing the misery a family experienced in a new home. Over the course of seven years, the mother made several hundred doctor and emergency room visits with her three children, seeking medication for infections, allergies, and asthma. The builder had forgotten to install a hole for the dryer vent. The hose from the dryer went into the wall behind the machine, but there was no place for the air and moisture to exit the building. Moisture from many loads of laundry poured into the insulated wall cavity and soaked it. Mold grew inside the wall, and whenever the dryer was used the exhaust air blew through the moldy insulation and back into the house, carrying spores into the air the family breathed. As soon as they discovered the cause of their illnesses the family moved out, leaving behind all their furniture and even their Christmas presents. The children's health improved immediately.

In another home I was inspecting the attic. The front of the house faced south and the rear faced north. When I looked at the south-facing roof sheathing, the plywood looked fine. On the north side it was a different story. The sheathing was soaking wet, and water was dripping from the tips of all the shingle nails protruding through it to the inside of the attic.

The owner had three children and had just done her fourth load of laundry for the day. A year earlier the family had finished the basement, and to save money their plumber suggested they vent the dryer into a lint trap in a closet under the basement stairs. Warm, moist air from the closet was less dense than cooler air and thus rose around plumbing pipes directly to the unheated attic, where vapor condensed onto the cooler, sunless north side of the roof. Fortunately this condensation had been occurring for only a year; had it gone on for two or three years more, the entire roof structure on the north side would have rotted.

Builders too are driven by economic considerations. One property I inspected was a spacious, newly renovated million dollar duplex basement condominium. The living room, dining room, and kitchen were on the upper level. The bedrooms were below, with direct access to a private city garden. Faucets were gleaming, carpets were plush, and the appliances were all top of the line. To vent the dryer to the outside, though, the builder would have had to go through a brick wall. To avoid this expense he vented the dryer into a small storage area under the front masonry stairs. To handle the excess moisture, he included a dehumidifier as a feature in the price of the condominium. The dehumidifier drained into a sewer ejection system (into which the toilets also drained), but it was leaking. The home buyers were getting some features they hadn't expected!

Cold Venting

Dryers should not be vented for great lengths through cold spaces. I was in the four-car garage of an expensive seven-year-old house in which the laundry was next to the garage. The dryer had to be vented at the opposite gable end of the garage. The many sections of metal vent pipe rested on the joists above the garage ceiling and traveled through an unheated attic. The warm, moist air from the dryer cooled as it traveled through the piping. As water condensed inside the pipes, it leaked out the joints and dripped onto the garage ceiling and down the rear walls, creating stains about every six feet where the sections of pipe connected.

From another investigator I heard about a similar situation where a flexible dryer vent hose went through an unheated attic. The hose drooped and formed loops inside the bays between the ceiling joists. Again, water condensed within the hose as the moist air traveling through it cooled. This type of plastic hose is watertight, so instead of leaking out the moisture formed puddles at the bottom of each loop. The lint provided nutrients for mold growth in each of these little ponds, so when the machine was not running air carrying mold spores backdrafted through the dryer and into the house, aggravating the owners' allergies.

Heated Venting

Occasionally a water heater or boiler will be placed next to a dryer in a small mechanical closet. In such an arrangement, the dryer can cause backdrafting if the closet has a solid door and there is no other source of makeup air. In one such mechanical closet with the door shut, I tested for combustion spillage with my TIF 8800 combustible gas detector at the vent pipe of a water heater. When the dryer was off there was normal draft at the vent pipe; but when the dryer was running it sucked the makeup air it needed from the water heater's vent pipe, and combustion gases filled the closet. In the best of all worlds, dryers should not be placed in small spaces next to combustion equipment. If you have such an arrangement in your home, a louvered door will supply air to eliminate the backdrafting.

I investigated a home for a man who was chemically sensitive. The recently renovated master bathroom contained an unvented gas dryer and an air return for the heating and cooling system. Summer and winter, when the dryer and the blower were operating simultaneously, combustion products, fabric softener, and lint were circulated throughout the condominium. I encountered a similar situation involving allergies in another single-family home. The first thing I noted when I entered was that the house smelled like a laundromat. We pulled the dryer away from the first-floor wall and discovered that the exhaust hose took an unusual route. Instead of venting directly to the outside through a wall, the hose had been fed through a hole in the floor. Unfortunately the return duct for the heating and cooling system was directly below the hole in the basement ceiling (the floor of the first level). This hadn't stopped the installer from cutting holes for the dryer hose through the top and bottom of the return duct. The hose then exited the building from the basement.

In this case the exhaust hose had become disconnected from the dryer. The holes in the floor and the sheet metal of the return duct were bigger than the hose itself, leaving gaps. Whenever the heat pump and the dryer operated simultaneously, air was sucked in through these gaps, creating airflow from the laundry room. Lint, fabric softener, and detergent chemicals exhausting directly from the dryer were drawn into the heating return and from there were circulating throughout the house.

To relieve his allergies the man had installed an expensive electronic air cleaner, but there was so much debris in the air that the electronic power module for the cleaner had burned out several times. He had also replaced the air conditioning compressor twice because the evaporator coil had clogged with lint.

Air-Drying

Some of us hang our clothes inside or outside to air-dry. In families with allergies, clothing should be dried only where the air is not full of allergens. Be careful to avoid moldy basements or pollen-laden trees. And a word of caution: it's a fire hazard to hang clothes within three feet of furnaces, boilers, or water heaters. Never use a boiler or furnace vent pipe to dry anything!

WASHING MACHINES

- Check your washing machine for leaks regularly and repair any you find.
- When the washing machine is not in use, close the water supply valves.
- Use water hoses covered with stainless steel.
- If the laundry room is not in the basement, consider installing a drain and waterproof flooring under the washer.
- Do not put a carpet on the floor of your laundry area.
- Avoid detergents that contain fabric softeners, fragrance, and enzymes.
- Don't let damp clothing sit around.
- If your washing machine develops an odor, clean any lint that may have accumulated around the base of the agitator or in the basket at the top.

DRYERS

- Don't use fabric softener sheets, particularly those with fragrance added.
- Always vent a dryer to the outside.
- Unless sloped correctly, dryer vent hoses should not travel for great lengths through cold spaces.
- Check to see that a dryer placed in a closet with combustion equipment doesn't cause backdrafting.
- Avoid placing a dryer in a mechanical closet that also contains the water heater or furnace. If you have such an arrangement, have a louvered door installed.
- Don't hang clothes to dry where there are allergens in the air.
- Keep the area near the flame of a gas dryer as lint-free as possible.

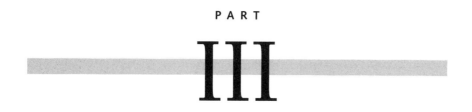

PART

III

Basements and Attics

Unfinished Basements

Like many people, you may not enjoy going down into your basement and breathing the air. But like it or not, basement air enters your lungs no matter where you are in the house. It's therefore vital to pay attention to its quality.

I was asked to investigate a two-hundred-year-old home because the owner had severe mold allergies and was suffering from sinus trouble and respiratory symptoms. The interior was one of the cleanest I had ever seen. There were hardwood floors with few rugs and furniture. Most people might consider this spartan, but because of her allergies to dust and mold, the woman believed this decor (or lack thereof) was necessary.

The basement was an entirely different story. One side of the basement developed a stream in heavy rain, and moldy leaves and other debris littered the whole basement and the attached crawl space. The house had steam heat, and pipes went from the basement and crawl space up to the radiators on the first floor. There were gaps around the pipes, and when the heat was on moldy warm air rose from the basement and crawl space into the rooms above. I demonstrated this air movement with a smoke pencil, which I use to track airflows. In this home I released puffs of smoke at cracks in the basement ceiling and in the gaps near the heat pipes. Standing on the first floor, the owner was enveloped in clouds of white smoke that billowed up through the openings. It was dramatic enough that she was convinced. Once the family cleaned the basement and crawl space and sealed the gaps around the pipes, her symptoms abated.

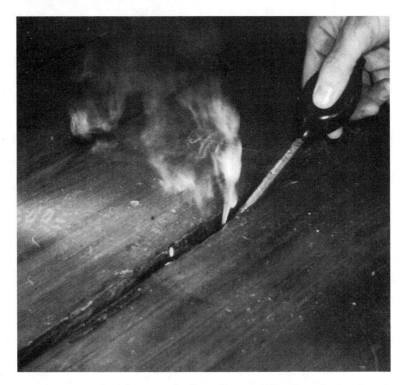

FIGURE 8.1. Smoke delineating the flow of basement air through a crack in a floor. Smoke from an air current tube illustrates the airflow from the basement through a crack in the living room floor of an older home with a very moldy basement. Though the upstairs was spotless the client, who was allergic to mold, suffered from constant symptoms.

Many air quality problems are caused by legions of unseen organisms growing in the basement. We don't necessarily think of the basement as part of the home, particularly if it's unfinished, but its conditions are intimately connected to the rest of a house. If the basement is teeming with life, by-products of biological growth will find their way into our living spaces. Although it's hard to believe, 30 to 50 percent of "fresh" house air, depending on the home and its construction, may come from the basement. Basement air travels by one route or another throughout the house, often carrying irritants with it.

CONTROLLING WATER ENTRY

There is a hidden ecology in a damp basement. Mildew grows on surfaces, and organisms such as mites and booklice feed on the mold. Spiders in turn dine on the hordes of crawling microscopic life. If you feel good about the drooping nets of spiderwebs hanging from your basement ceiling, think again.

Minimizing moisture in your basement is an important step to controlling microscopic plant and animal life. The most obvious source is external water that finds its way in, and the most common cause of entry is improper dispersal of roof water: gutters and grading, grading and gutters. When land slopes toward the house, water runs toward the foundation. In a heavy rain, moisture soaks into the soil at the foundation and can leak into the basement, particularly if there are cracks in the masonry walls. Proper handling of roof and grade water is particularly important with older stone foundations, which are often full of gaps. If you have a stone foundation, it's a good idea to keep the mortar intact. No matter what kind of foundation you have, clogged or missing gutters make the problem worse by allowing water to pond close to the house. (For further discussion of gutters and grading, see chapter 15, on the exterior of the home.)

A quick way to see if roof or grade water is entering is to flood the area near a downspout very close to the foundation with water from a hose, then go into the basement to see if water comes in. On a few inspections I have done just such testing. In one home I turned the hose on and asked the broker to go into the basement and shout when water began to appear. I heard him scream as soon as he went down the stairs. A little sooner than I expected, a sizable puddle had formed in the corner, under the oil tank. The heavily rusted tank legs spoke silently of numerous earlier baths.

Sump pumps can help control basement water, especially in areas with a high water table. Wherever you live, the water table is somewhere below your house. It may be twenty feet down or twenty inches, or even one inch below the basement floor slab. If you dig a hole and the bottom fills with water, you've reached the water table. Above the water table the spaces between the soil particles are filled with air and water vapor; below it they are filled with liquid water. The layer above the water table, where there is air and vapor in the soil, is called the vadose zone. People prefer to have their foundations in the vadose zone rather than below the water table, but sometimes topography disappoints us.

The sump pump keeps a high water table beneath the top of the floor slab. (A sump is the hole in the floor, and the pump empties the water from the sump.) A pump should be kept low enough to prevent water from overflowing the sump. It should not be placed too low, however, for if there is a high water table the pump will run continuously, creating a water dispersal headache and using too much electrical power. The motor may also burn out more frequently with constant use.

One woman who lived near a lake had this problem with her pump, which was at the bottom of the sump, under approximately two feet of water. The pump ran almost continuously, discharging water through a long hose that ran over the lawn to the curb. Where the water flowed out, the curb and asphalt were wet, and the pavement was green with algae. The water table was high, so every house on that side of the street had a similar hose across its lawn. Hers was the only "green river," however, because none of her neighbors had their pumps positioned as low as she did. I explained that she should raise her pump, since the level of the water table in her basement was about the same as the lake. She was trying to empty the entire lake that bordered all the yards on her side of the street.

Some people depend too readily on sump pumps instead of taking care of the underlying condition. For example, I inspected another home with a sump pump that was operating frequently. As soon as the pump drained the sump, water rushed back in. At first I thought the water table was high, but this wasn't the case. Even though all the fixtures were off and the water meter dial was motionless, I noticed a peculiar hissing noise in the vicinity of the water main. I recommended that the seller inform the town water department. A representative discovered that the city water main was broken in the street and that millions of gallons of water had been lost. Coincidentally, when the city main was fixed, five neighbors were also able to disconnect their sump pumps because they no longer had water in their basements.

I've found some strange things, including frogs, in basement sumps. Some items like dead mice, moldy toilet paper, and other biodegradable debris can be a source of air quality problems. Keep your sump clean and install a nonbiodegradable cover that can be easily removed for periodic checks. If there are high radon levels in the soil, the sump can also be a source of radon gas in the basement, and you may have to install an airtight radon cover (see "Radon Gas" later in this chapter).

When the pump operates, be sure no water squirts out of the pipes or splashes out of the sump. In one home the sump pump was housed in a closet. Near the end of the discharge cycle, water squirted out of the weep hole and splashed onto the drywall. All the walls of the closet were covered with *Stachybotrys,* a potentially toxic mold.

A last caution about sump pumps. If your system depends on electricity, never assume it will always work. Very often, power failures occur during heavy storms, and you lose your electricity precisely when you need it most. If you depend heavily on a sump pump to keep your basement dry, consider installing a battery-operated backup pump. If you are in a rural area, you may want to have a power generator on hand, because batteries don't last very long. Never operate a gasoline engine indoors; you could be asphyxiated from the exhaust while trying to keep your basement from drowning.

BASEMENT RAIN FORESTS

Surprising as it may seem, humidity and condensation rather than leaks or flooding cause most basement mold I see. For example, water that condenses on uninsulated cold water pipes or on a pressure tank associated with well water storage can drip onto the floor or soak into stored goods. If the pipes in your basement sweat like this, installing foam insulation around them will prevent condensation. Insulation for copper pipes comes in various diameters to fit most common pipe sizes.

In most basements, foundation masonry (stone, brick, concrete blocks, or poured concrete) is cooler than the upstairs walls and floor; during the summer it is often below the dew point of the basement air, and moisture will condense on the masonry and even on goods stored close to or touching it.

Whatever type of foundation you have, the masonry surfaces acquire a layer of house dust. Dust collects even on vertical walls, for several reasons. First, microscopic plant fibers, such as cellulose from sawdust and lint, adhere to the rough wall surface. As airflows carry other particles over the cellulose fibers, suspended biodegradable particles (such as skin scales and pollen) collide with them and stick. Second, spiders are constantly traversing foundation walls, foraging for insects. They leave a trail of fine silk that dust can stick to. When I look under the microscope at surface samples I take with sticky tape, I'm always amazed to see vast networks of spider silk.

Biodegradable dust accumulates on the floors and walls, and many foundation walls are also covered with at least a fine layer of mold or actinomycetes (soil organisms) growing on the dust, though these may not become airborne unless they are disturbed. Eventually every particle of biodegradable dust that lands on basement masonry will probably be consumed by some living organism, particularly if the relative humidity is high. (To avoid this ecological progression, see "Drying Out" later in this chapter.)

Foundation walls and floors that are painted and smooth are easier to keep clean. Surfaces can be vacuumed with a HEPA vacuum cleaner or disinfected with diluted bleach (or both), though care must be taken not to stir up irritating dust during cleaning. Dirt floors, on the other hand, can never be cleaned. A significant percentage of soil consists of living organisms, and their digestive enzymes are poised to receive the nutrients we shed. With a ready food source and adequate soil moisture, mold and other microorganisms will proliferate. If you have a moldy dirt floor in your basement, *I urge you to have a contractor install a concrete floor over a vapor barrier and crushed stone* (under containment conditions).

Fiberglass Canopy

Many basements have exposed fiberglass ceiling insulation between the joists for the first floor; unfortunately, some building codes even require insulation. The fiberglass acts as a filter and can accumulate significant amounts of biodegradable dust and allergens. In approximately one-third of the sick homes with exposed fiberglass basement insulation that I have inspected, and in nearly all the crawl spaces, moisture levels had at some point been excessive, and vast populations of fungi and mites were growing in ceiling fiberglass insulation that looked clean. If there are pets in the home, then the fiberglass sometimes contains dander, which besides being an allergen is also mold fodder.

If dusty insulation becomes damp from condensation or a pipe leak, mold will have the moisture it needs to grow. Once a mold spore germinates, it sends

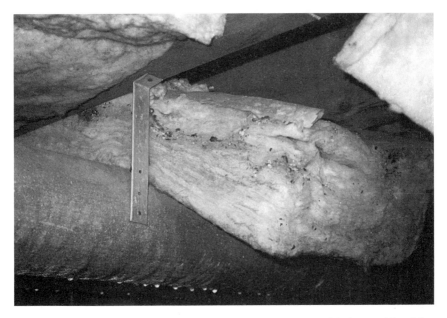

FIGURE 8.2. Wet, dirty insulation. When the weather turned quickly from cold and dry to warm and humid, condensed water dripped from various surfaces in the basement, including the fiberglass insulation and metal heat duct. Under these conditions, mold spores start to germinate. Mouse droppings (the dark dots) in the insulation were covered with blue-green *Penicillium* mold, suggesting that such dew point conditions had happened before.

out hyphae that travel along the glass fibers and digest any adhering particulates they encounter. Mold-eating mites move in thereafter to dine on the spores and hyphae. When people walk on the floors above moldy insulation, or when work is done on basement piping or electrical wiring, the fiberglass fibers are disturbed and become airborne, along with clouds of particulates containing whatever allergens are present. Fiberglass insulation that is contaminated in this fashion can be extremely difficult to identify as a source of indoor air quality problems.

Installing fiberglass insulation with the vapor barrier side (usually tar paper) down will prevent biodegradable dust from accumulating in the fiberglass, but it will not stop the paper in the barrier from getting moldy if moisture condenses in the material. I recommend installing a noncombustible covering, such as drywall, over fiberglass insulation in a basement ceiling.

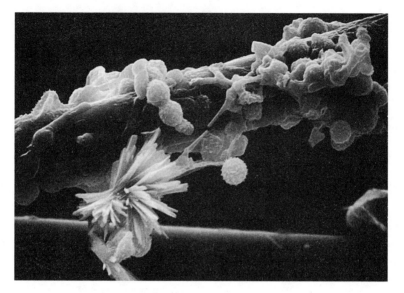

FIGURE 8.3. Two fiberglass fibers, one covered with mold hyphae and spores. The wheel of needles between the two fibers probably consists of crystallized waste products produced by the mold as it digests the house dust settled on the fiber. When contaminated fiberglass insulation in a basement ceiling is disturbed even slightly, thousands of spores become airborne. (2,000× SEM)

(Mold will still grow on drywall paper if the relative humidity is high enough.) Don't install clear, exposed polyethylene vapor barrier: it is combustible and can ignite if it touches an incandescent lightbulb.

You never know what you will find in uncovered basement insulation. One couple was looking for a house where the wife could have a basement office. They found one they liked very much. The basement was unfinished but roomy, and the ceiling was already insulated with exposed fiberglass. The wife noticed on their first visit that there was a litter box in the basement. She was very allergic to cats, and the sellers had two. The couple decided to buy the house anyway, and after the closing but before they moved in, they asked me what they would have to do to renovate the basement space.

There was evidence of moisture in the basement, but I was more concerned about cat dander that might have accumulated in the dust in the fiberglass ceiling. I recommended they take out all the old insulation and use a HEPA vacuum to clean the joists and subfloor, then lightly spray paint the accessible wood structure before beginning the renovation. In fact, given her sensitivity to cat allergens, I encouraged them to take these steps before moving into the house.

The couple made a deal. The husband would remove and bag the insulation, and the wife (wearing an N95 NIOSH fine-particle mask for protection) would clean the floor. On the hottest day of the summer, they began their work. The next day the wife called to report their progress. She described areas where so many mouse droppings had fallen from the insulation that the concrete floor was barely visible. When she walked across the masonry, her feet crunched mouse skeletons swaddled in fiberglass. When I wondered aloud how such a widespread mouse infestation was possible with two cats living in the house, she replied that they must have been lazy. And I was worried about cat dander!

In another home the owner had suffered allergy symptoms for three years, ever since moving into the house. When she was exposed to air from the basement she developed rashes. She kept the basement scrupulously clean, but she naturally avoided entering it as much as possible, even though the walls and floor were painted and no items were stored there. The flows from the hot-air heating system also bothered her, so she placed stockings on some registers as filters and kept others closed. When the blower was operating, the stockings restricted the airflow to such an extent that air was pouring out of all the duct joints into the basement, increasing the air pressure there and disturbing the dust in the fiberglass. At the first-floor level the air pressure was reduced because the single large return was pulling air into the system and there was an insufficient supply of corresponding air from the blocked registers.

In this home two forces were moving air up from the basement: the excess air pressure in the basement and the reduced pressure on the first floor. When I smoke tested the airflows, I found that air from the basement rushed through large gaps under the basement door and around the tub and pipe openings in the bathroom. The basement ceiling was insulated with fiberglass that was full of mold and mites, and the allergens were carried upstairs by the airflows. The owner had a professional remove the basement insulation, and the ceiling structure was lightly spray painted to contain surface dust. She removed the stockings from the heat registers, had the furnace and ducts cleaned, and added an efficient filter. Within a week her rashes disappeared.

The air that flows into and out of a home's blower system must be balanced: for every cubic foot of air distributed to all the rooms, one cubic foot of air must be drawn in by the system return. When a system is not balanced, as is often the case, trouble can result.

Stored Goods

Possessions stored in a basement that is damp from condensation, leaks, or flooding can become contaminated, particularly if the items touch foundation walls or the floor. When paper goods, such as boxes or newspapers, rest directly on concrete, mold often grows at the bottom. This type of growth is helped along by floor water from leaks, but it can spread even without such leaks. Unless the mold grows up the sides, you may not be aware of its presence. When I notice rectangular black shapes on a floor—residues outlining moldy items that have been removed—I avoid stepping on them, since they may contain *Stachybotrys* mold. When people do step on such spots, mold spores and other microscopic bits of contaminated debris are disturbed and become airborne.

A physician referred one client to me after a lung biopsy revealed that the man's very reduced lung capacity was due to hypersensitivity pneumonitis. This pulmonary condition, characterized by immune inflammation in the lungs, is sometimes caused by chronic exposure to mold spores and other bioaerosols. The man owned a very large collection of classical records that were stored in a damp, moldy basement. After he retired his wife suggested he reorganize his collection and thin it out because it took up too much basement space. He spent several hours a day over two or three years reviewing his beloved albums, sorting them into "sell" and "keep" categories while exposing his lungs to mold spores from the fungi growing on the album covers. The couple had to get rid of all the moldy record covers and books and have the foundation walls professionally cleaned and the basement ceiling structure spray painted.

I recommend storing as little as possible in basements. To protect items against moisture from condensation, leaks, and flooding, never place possessions up against the basement walls or directly on the floor—a common practice. Items stored in unfinished basements should be on shelves (preferably metal or plastic) at least two feet from the foundation walls and a few inches above the floor. You can raise things on pallets of pressure-treated wood resting on bricks or concrete blocks (untreated wood pallets can become moldy). Storing items off the floor will also keep them dry if your basement gets a few inches of water in a storm.

Storing clothing and other fabric items in airtight plastic boxes or bags will help protect them from excessive basement humidity. One caution, though: don't put fabric in airtight containers during humid weather. Moisture is adsorbed (bound to the surface of the fibers) before it is absorbed (trapped as liquid between the fibers). At 100 percent relative humidity a cotton shirt may weigh about 28 percent more than it does when the air is very dry because individual water molecules in the air are adsorbed by the cellulose fibers. At every level of relative humidity (except zero), adsorbed moisture will be present. When many individual water molecules (not in ice) are joined together, they behave as a liquid; when they are separated from each other and bound to a surface, they behave as if they are part of the surface they are bonded to, so a cotton shirt carrying 28 percent of its weight in adsorbed water may still feel dry.

Cotton cloth that is dripping wet has first adsorbed and then absorbed moisture. The adsorbed water will still be present when most of the absorbed water has been squeezed out, because it takes more energy to break the bond between the water molecule and the cellulose than to wring out the liquid water.

If you pack a shirt that feels dry into a plastic bag on a humid day, the adsorbed moisture will remain in the bag. As the room cools, the moisture may condense on the material or on the plastic, and if spores are present mold may grow. If you must pack away clothing on humid days, place the articles in the dryer first. Cotton fresh from a hot dryer will have a very low moisture content, but if the material is allowed to remain in humid air, moisture will again be adsorbed onto the fibers. If possible, therefore, pack the clothing while it is still warm.

If you experience a significant basement flood, discard stored items that have absorbed water, such as mattresses and sofas. Replace any cardboard boxes that have become wet, because mold spores can germinate within hours. Be extremely careful about using large-volume fans to dry the basement; in an already moldy basement they can blow spores around and create significant air quality problems.

It takes far less moisture than a flood to cause trouble. For example, a family purchased a home with a very damp basement. They thought it would be safe to put all their winter clothing in a large cedar closet in the basement, but when they went to retrieve their clothing in the fall it was covered with *Aspergillus* mold. The relative humidity in the closet was no different from that in the rest of the basement, and though the odor of cedar may repel insects, it did not slow the mold down in the least.

For those who are highly sensitized, mold exposure can even be deadly. Another family who called me for help also had a damp basement, and all their stored goods were covered with mold. The family's teenage daughter was experiencing anaphylaxis; she would go into shock and stop breathing, generally in the middle of the night. The cause of her illness was unknown. Her parents kept an extra mattress in her bedroom, and every night one of them kept vigil after she had fallen asleep. The cat's litter box was in the basement, and the door was left open so the animal could go up and down freely. Airflows were carrying the mold contamination from the basement up into the living spaces.

I recommended the family install a pet door to the basement and hire a professional cleaning firm. Because the girl might have been sensitized to the basement dust, the workers did all they could to prevent disturbed dust from rising into the rest of the house. This extraordinary effort, similar in scope to an asbestos mitigation, entailed covering all the floors at the first level with plastic, gasketing the basement door, and sealing gaps around all the pipes that rose to the upper levels. The company also created negative pressure by blowing HEPA-filtered air out through a basement window. This way, even if there were any small openings left unsealed between the basement and the first floor, air would flow into the basement rather than the other way around. To be safe, the daughter also stayed out of the house until all the rooms had been thoroughly cleaned with a HEPA vacuum (see chapter 14).

I later heard that the girl, who had been hospitalized at least three times in the months before the cleanup, needed no hospitalization afterward.

DUCT CONVEYANCE

I was called by one condominium owner who told me she could smell mold in her unit on the third floor of a ninety-year-old building with hot-air heat. This seemed curious, since it's unusual to have mold odor on the top floor of a building. When I walked into her unit, I readily agreed about the strong mold odor, which seemed to be coming out of one of her heat ducts.

We went into the basement and determined that the duct leading to that register passed through the ceiling of a storage area belonging to another unit owner. The basement had flooded several times because of sewer backups, and all the stored goods were covered with mold. The odor in the storage area was overpowering—a stronger version of the smell on the third floor.

In houses heated by hot-air systems, there can be a constant "passive" (convective) airflow through the entire duct system even when the blower is off. Flows from the basement to the other rooms can be increased if the ducts leak. When the heat was off, air from the storage area was drawn into the system by convection through the space in the chase (vertical shaft) around the heat duct and several gaps in the loose duct joint. The odor disappeared when the moldy furniture was removed and the duct and chase were sealed.

I went to another home, more modest and newer, where the parents were very concerned because their young son had been experiencing chronic fevers and had been hospitalized numerous times. The child had been taking antibiotics for months to no avail. There was a hot-air heating system in the home, and the damp basement was packed full of furniture acquired from yard sales. They had biodegradable items sitting directly on the floor and up against the foundation walls. Everything was covered with visible mildew from *Cladosporium* growth.

The bottom of the furnace air return had never been secured properly, so there was a large gap. When the heating system was operating, mold spores from the basement were sucked in and blown upstairs with the hot air. With a Burkard sampler, I measured the largest concentration of spores I had ever seen—about 300,000 *Cladosporium* spores per cubic meter of air—coming out of the heat register in the boy's bedroom. There were other problems in the home as well. Three of my recommendations were to install a bottom at the return cabinet, eliminate the moldy furniture, and improve the grading around the foundation so less water would enter the basement.

Another client, referred by her pulmonologist, had been suffering from hypersensitivity pneumonitis (HP). Because she became breathless so readily, she had been basically housebound for three years. Her house was at the bottom of a hill and also had a basement garage with a driveway that sloped sharply down from the street. The house backed up to a swamp, so the water table was high. All these factors conspired against the client, for during heavy summer rains the basement flooded, sometimes with as much as twelve inches of water. Mold growth in the basement was extensive, and the hot-air heating system was helping to circulate spores throughout the living spaces.

The woman's physician had already ordered a lab test on her blood serum for reactivity to molds (an HP screen), and it showed a mildly elevated level of IgE (immunoglobulin E) in reaction to one type of *Aspergillus* mold. I took Andersen air samples in the home and shipped the petri dishes overnight to the same lab for additional testing, which indicated the woman had *very* elevated levels of IgE in reaction to the specific species of *Aspergillus* growing in her home.

The client had a professional thoroughly clean the basement and the heating system, and her respiratory capacity went from 50 percent of normal to 100 percent.

DRYING OUT

Even if it is unfinished, a basement should be kept as dry as possible to keep mold growth and insect populations at a minimum. Relative humidity should be below 50 percent. People who realize how important it is to reduce basement moisture operate dehumidifiers, but in most homes where they are in use I still find problems.

For example, the dehumidifier coil can be full of biological growth. The coils, particularly a spiral configuration, accumulate a layer of dust that is kept constantly wet by the condensation. If you cut wood in the basement, your dehumidifier can trap lots of sawdust. Mold, bacteria, and other organisms grow on cellulose as well as on other types of dust. Check the cooling coils on your dehumidifier regularly and be sure there is no biological slime clinging to them. If there is, the machine itself can disperse airborne irritants. Contam-

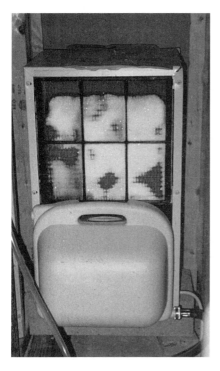

FIGURE 8.4. Basement dehumidifier left operating in the winter. Because there was so little moisture, the cooling coils stayed below the freezing point of water, and what little moisture did condense froze on the coil. The dirty filter was stuck in the ice layer. When the ice melted, dust on the filter no doubt became moldy.

inated coils can be cleaned with a sprayer and a brush (do this outside). Refer to the manufacturer's cleaning directions, and do not wet any electrical components.

I also find that people don't empty the drain buckets of their dehumidifiers often enough. Most dehumidifiers stop running when the bucket is full, defeating their purpose. In addition, any biodegradable debris inside the bucket will fester. In humid conditions the drain bucket sometimes has to be emptied two or three times a day. One way to avoid this annoying chore is to suspend the dehumidifier above a basement sink and let the water drain directly into it through a garden hose. If you don't have a basement sink, you can purchase a small condensate pump (sold for use in air conditioning systems) and pump the water outside through a plastic tube. If you want to use either of these means, be sure to buy a dehumidifier with a hose fitting on the condensate tray.

A dehumidifier should be operated in a clean basement, or the air movement the machine generates can disturb and disperse irritating dust. In addition, don't operate a dehumidifier during the winter, when the air is dry, or when the temperature is below 65°F. If the compressor is running but there is little or no water condensing (or if the coils are iced over), you are wasting your money.

Another wasteful mistake homeowners make is to keep the basement windows open when they operate dehumidifiers. This is like trying to dehumidify the air in the whole neighborhood. It's similarly wasteful to leave the door to the rest of the house open. The only way to successfully dehumidify the basement is to isolate it from the outside and from the rest of the house. If a basement consists of several rooms or of isolated areas such as storage closets, keep the connecting doors open or use more than one dehumidifier.

I recommend purchasing an expensive and efficient dehumidifier, which will have about three times the capacity of most less expensive models and also a very efficient media filter to prevent biodegradable dust from accumulating on the moist cooling coils (see the resource guide at the end of the book). No matter what model you choose, the only way to know if your dehumidifier is doing its job is to measure the basement's relative humidity. This means buying a hygrometer, which can be purchased in most hardware stores.

CRAWL SPACES

Some homes or additions are built over crawl spaces—shallow spaces between the ground and floor structure—rather than full basements. Although in some parts of the country crawl spaces are common, I would never choose to live in a home with one because I have seen them cause so many problems. In addition, very few people who have crawl spaces think of dehumidifying them. I discourage anyone with allergies or asthma from purchasing such a home unless the crawl space is spotless and has concrete floors and walls. Crawl spaces with dirt floors make me shudder.

I inspected an apartment for a tenant who was paying a substantial rent for his exclusive unit but had never been able to live there because the air had a foul odor that made his allergies worse. The first-floor apartment was directly above a sandy crawl space with two sources of unwelcome water. First, the downspouts dumped water directly at the foundation wall rather than directing it away from the building. When it rained, water seeped through the foundation and formed meandering streams that ran through the crawl space.

Second, there was a pond of sewage seven feet across and six inches deep at the bottom of a concrete sump that contained the uncapped clean-out for the building sewer system. In addition, rodent burrows lined several of the sand mounds near the sump.

Meanwhile, in the luxury unit above, I vacuumed the living room carpeting with a special filter cassette to obtain a sample of dust so I could quantify dust mite allergens. I also observed the material in the cassette with a low-power microscope and was astonished to see a silverfish scurrying after six fleeing dust mites. It was the first time I had ever seen dust mites crawl out of their habitat; usually they stay hidden in the dust for protection. In this case they were being chased by the silverfish, searching frantically for its next meal. It was the food chain on a microscopic level, all sucked from an apartment carpet!

I believe this living jungle was caused by the elevated moisture conditions in the crawl space below. Moisture saturated the air in the crawl space as well as the wood framing, the flooring, and the carpeting above. Insects thrived in the high humidity in the carpet. In addition, an unwelcome smell rose into the apartment from the sewage pond in the crawl space. The tenant used the evidence of the damp stench as well as my report to break his lease.

Another desperate homeowner asked me to inspect the crawl space under his five-year-old dining room addition. The previous day he had stood outside by the crawl space ventilation louver and heard water dripping, though he could not recall having any plumbing installed in the room above. He had not looked into the crawl space in five years.

The crawl space was above grade, and when I removed the access vent and looked inside I could not believe my eyes. White and tan tendrils of fungal hyphae (mycelium) hung from every joist, and dark stains covered the wall framing. The soil was damp, and there was an odor of mold. What was the source of moisture? The architect had not wanted to put gutters on the addition, and the builder neglected to put a vapor barrier over the soil. Moisture from the damp soil evaporated into the space.

The most extraordinary part of this scene was not the fungus but the main beam. Although it superficially appeared satisfactory, it was cracked from top to bottom at the center of its longest span. The man told me he had held a party for thirty guests the weekend before. The load of all of these people had cracked the beam, weakened by the unseen decay. Miraculously, it had not failed. Later that day, when I told the builder about the crack, he was so concerned the addition might collapse that he rushed over to support the beam with concrete blocks. I heard from another builder about an addition that had failed within three years owing to fungal growth caused by excessive moisture in a crawl space.

Most building codes require that crawl spaces be ventilated to the exterior. In many climates, however, these vents allow in more moisture than they "ventilate." Vapor barriers on the soil, which are also required by many building codes, are a very important way to minimize crawl space moisture and biological growth. Unfortunately, vapor barriers are often torn or disrupted by careless homeowners or contractors who enter the crawl space to do work. To be effective, a vapor barrier must be airtight. I prefer a dehumidified crawl space that is closed to the outside and has a vapor barrier or concrete floor. Conditions in a crawl space should be monitored. Make a point of regularly looking in. Keep a hygrometer there, and if the relative humidity rises above 70 percent, expect to find mold growth and a need for improvements. Try to keep the relative humidity below 50 percent.

Crawl Space Pets and Pests

I have been called to look at many homes with powerful unpleasant odors, often originating in crawl spaces. Typically the sources are mold or pest infestations in fiberglass ceiling insulation or else animal excrement and other biodegradable debris in the soil. In some homes the odor will be apparent upstairs even when there is no visible connection between the crawl space and the interior.

One couple thought they had a powerful mold odor coming from their basement. Although they did have significant flooding and mold there, the odor that concerned them originated in the dirt-floored crawl space. It turned out that while their daughter was on vacation they had offered to keep her cat. Apparently the cat preferred the crawl space to the litter box.

Crawl spaces also attract wild animals. Fiberglass insulation can be an attractive nesting site for bees. Even framing openings that aren't large enough to be noticed can provide access for small rodents. Some of these animals would rather nest in open fiberglass insulation than in a log or elsewhere in the wild. Mice urinate and defecate inside the fiberglass, and if they die there the smell is even worse.

An insurance agent purchased a single-family home to use for offices. The house had not been well maintained, and after he bought the property he had to clean the basement and crawl space very thoroughly to eliminate mold. Although he spent a great deal of money, a lingering odor persisted. The crawl space ceiling insulation was covered with a plastic vapor barrier, and I could see brown stains and liquid from rodent infestations. After the insulation was eliminated and the joists spray painted, the odor disappeared.

Because crawl spaces are often damp and inaccessible, they may harbor termites. In one home treated for termites, the applicator sprayed pesticide on the soil in the crawl space as well as on the floor joists. This type of "broadcast" spraying is not permitted. In this case some of the framing in the crawl space was covered with chlordane, a particularly persistent, odorous, semi-volatile toxic chemical, which evaporated into the basement and moved with airflows into the upper levels of the house. One of the owners was a nurse who was chemically sensitive. She could no longer work in the hospital, where she had already been exposed to numerous chemicals and irritants. As is so often the case, her home provided no respite.

Though this is an extreme case of an overzealous and inappropriate application of a powerful pesticide, even when the chemicals are correctly and appropriately applied they can enter the house air through a dirt floor in a crawl space. This is another reason I feel strongly that dirt floors in crawl spaces should be sealed with crushed stone, vapor barrier, and concrete.

RADON GAS

In some areas of the country, the levels of radon (a radioactive, carcinogenic gas) in the soil are high. Radon can enter a basement from a sump, particularly if a system of piping to collect subslab water is connected to the sump. An airtight plastic sump cover may reduce radon entry. Radon also enters a basement with other soil gases through dirt floors and cracks in masonry floors and walls. These flows occur because the pressure inside the house is usually less than that of the gases in the soil. Elevated radon levels are a particular concern if people spend time in the basement. Even if the basement isn't used much, air with radon can enter the upper floors. In general the level of radon on the first floor is one-half to one-third that in the basement—proof again that we inevitably breathe basement air upstairs.

A radon mitigation system draws soil gases, including radon, out of the spaces that surround a basement foundation and floor slab. A plastic pipe is sunk into crushed stone in the soil beneath the basement floor. The pipe rises through the house and into the attic, where an in-line (axial) fan secured to the pipe draws the radon-containing air from the soil behind the basement masonry and blows the radioactive gas out above the roof, where it dissipates.

I was walking around the outside of one home when I heard a throaty hum. After searching high and low, I finally discovered that a plastic pipe exiting the roof was the source of the noise. The pipe was part of a radon mitigation system. The potential buyer was very concerned about cancer and radon gas. She had previously withdrawn an offer on another property because test results had uncovered an elevated radon level in the basement.

In this house the sellers had installed a radon mitigation system but had never informed the real estate agent or the buyer that it existed. All the piping in the basement was concealed by stored goods, and the exhaust fan I had heard from the outside had been walled in when the attic was renovated as a master bedroom. The system was operating, but there was no access to the fan for servicing. Again, the buyer declined to purchase the home.

Unlike most unhealthful particles and gases in air, radon gas cannot be smelled or tasted, and it causes no immediate symptoms. In fact a liter of air with radon and one without it are nearly identical in every way, because at the action level of four picocuries of radon per liter of air suggested by the Environmental Protection Agency (EPA), only about one atom in 30,000,000,000,000,000,000 in a liter of air is radon! Yet radioactive atoms are so dangerous that even if inhaled at this concentration, they increase the risk of lung cancer. If you smoke and have elevated radon in your home, your likelihood of having lung cancer rises.

Every home therefore should be tested for radon as recommended by the EPA. Radon test kits are inexpensive and easy to use. If the concentration in the lowest lived-in level is above four picocuries per liter, additional testing or mitigation may be needed. Mitigation systems generally cost under $2,000 and are worth the investment to protect your health and property. If you have a mitigation system in your house, remember to maintain it and to disclose its presence to any prospective buyers.

Do not install a system yourself; seek a licensed contractor. I inspected a house where the seller had installed a radon exhaust fan in his basement and connected it to a dryer hose that discharged beneath the rear deck. The connection at the interior was loose, and radon-laden air poured into the basement. In addition, the discharge beneath the deck enveloped his barbecue and his daughter's sandbox in radioactive gas.

BASEMENT ACTIVITIES

It's tempting to expand certain activities into a basement, such as children's play or adults' exercise. I don't recommend this, however, because basement dust tends to be contaminated with mold spores and insect fecal allergens (see chapter 9). Particularly for people who have allergies or asthma, spending extended time in contaminated spaces can lead to respiratory distress. To make matters worse, both play and exercise raise respiration rates and disturb dust, both of which can increase the severity of exposure and symptoms. I realize it's often convenient to do laundry in basements: if they are kept clean of dust and adequately dehumidified, this should not pose an excessive risk.

RECOMMENDATIONS

WATER ENTRY

- Be sure grading around the house leads water away from the foundation.
- Water from downspouts should be discharged away from the foundation.
- Test your foundation by running a hose in the area where you suspect a leak.

- Keep a sump pump low enough to prevent overflow from your sump during heavy rain, but don't keep it submerged below the water table so that it runs almost continuously.
- If necessary, get a battery-operated backup sump pump.
- Immediately discard items such as sofas and mattresses that have been soaked.
- Use caution when drying out flooded basements. If there is basement mold, fans can make asthma symptoms worse.

STORED GOODS

- Store goods on pallets or shelving away from foundation walls and floor.
- Minimize basement storage of possessions.
- Seal clothing in plastic to protect it from mildew, but only when the item itself is dry or when relative humidity is under 30 percent.

MOISTURE AND HUMIDITY

- Insulate cold water pipes in humid areas to prevent sweating.
- Maintain basement relative humidity under 50 percent.
- Use a dehumidifier, but keep it and the basement dust-free.
- If possible, drain a dehumidifier into a sink or use a condensate pump to dispose of condensed water.
- If you have multiple rooms in your basement, use a ducted dehumidifier.
- Keep basements and crawl spaces as dry as possible. If there are leaks in pipes, repair them. If water is condensing on surfaces, determine the cause and eliminate it.

CRAWL SPACES

- Dehumidify rather than ventilate.
- Monitor conditions in a crawl space regularly. Keep relative humidity under 50 percent.

- Do all you can to keep all pests and pets out of a crawl space.
- If you note a strong chemical odor in a crawl space, have the space investigated. Research the history of the house to see if the building has ever been treated for pests.

RADON

- Test your basement and the rest of your home for radon. Follow EPA guidelines for testing.
- If radon is present, have a radon mitigation system installed by a licensed contractor.

MISCELLANEOUS

- In homes where highly sensitized individuals reside, mold cleanup and basement renovations should be undertaken by professionals using asbestos-level containment.
- Dirt floors, whether in basements or in crawl spaces, should be covered with concrete over crushed stone (where feasible) and a vapor barrier. Otherwise, keep soil free of all biodegradable materials and cover it with a heavy, airtight polyethylene vapor barrier.
- Keep basement floors and walls free of dust. If you are sensitized, always wear an N95 NIOSH fine-particle mask. Paint surfaces to make cleaning easier, but antifungal paint with mildewcide can off-gas and be irritating.
- Test old exposed fiberglass insulation for mold growth. If it is contaminated, have it professionally removed.
- Avoid using unfinished basements as if they were part of the living space in the house (as exercise or play areas, for example).
- Install a cat door if the litter box is in the basement.

Finished Basements

In my indoor air quality investigations, I have found that people with respiratory problems are almost twice as likely to be living in houses with finished, carpeted rooms below grade (below ground level) as in those without them. I hate to see people occupying such rooms because, as you will see from the stories that follow, most basements and other spaces below grade are not suited for use as playrooms, exercise rooms, and bedrooms.

In this chapter I concentrate on the IAQ problems caused by finished, below-grade rooms. Even if your basement is finished rather than unfinished, be sure to read chapter 8 as well, which contains information and suggestions relevant to all below-grade spaces.

LEAKS AND FLOODS

One young couple purchased a three-year-old house and, after living there a few months, decided to finish the basement. They installed walls, shelves, and carpeting and transformed the space into a family room, exercise room, and laundry area. That fall, during a heavy rain, a small amount of water leaked onto the floor from the bulkhead and soaked into a corner of the carpet under the treadmill. The wife, who was pregnant, went on maternity leave from her job in December. To keep fit, she set out on an exercise program in the basement. She subsequently experienced shortness of breath and was hospitalized; her doctors assumed that the pregnancy was causing her respiratory distress. After the child was born the woman renewed her exercise regimen. When she once more developed severe breathing difficulties as well as a dry cough, she was hospitalized again, and her doctors determined that her respiratory capacity was less than 70 percent of normal.

It became clear that her pregnancy had not been the cause of the condition. After she was diagnosed with hypersensitivity pneumonitis, she called me. With a Burkard sampler, I found that the concentration of spores of the *Penicillium-Aspergillus* type was about 50,000 per cubic meter of air (I consider a concentration of 1,000 spores per cubic meter to be high). It was no surprise that I also found extensive mold growth in the basement carpet dust. I suggested the woman stay out of the basement until it could be thoroughly cleaned by a professional. I also recommended vinyl flooring. Within months, her respiratory capacity returned to 100 percent.

In another potentially unhealthy situation, a physician called me after reading newspaper accounts of infants in Cleveland dying, possibly because of exposure to *Stachybotrys* mold. He and his wife had just brought their first baby home from the hospital, and he was worried about mold growth in his basement. They were renting, and when they first saw the home they had inquired about stains on the finished basement walls. The landlord claimed the basement had flooded only once.

When I looked carefully around the finished basement, I could see signs that flooding had occurred several times, most likely from sewer backups. I also wondered if mold was growing inside the walls. I tapped on the wall and took a Burkard air sample directly in front of an electrical outlet. The wall consisted of paneling over drywall, and by pushing on the panel (while wearing an N95 NIOSH mask), I forced air out from between the two layers. A cloud of white smoke appeared that I assumed was drywall dust. But when I looked at that sample under the microscope, it consisted of tens of thousands of *Penicillium* mold spores. Though I did not find *Stachybotrys* mold, nonetheless I encouraged the family to move.

I have inspected numerous basement apartments where water penetrated walls and leaked under doors. In one very expensive garden-level condominium, the basement master bedroom opened onto steps leading up to a private urban garden. The scene was bucolic. One could lie in bed and look through the glass sliding door onto a pastoral scene. Unfortunately, whenever it rained heavily water cascaded down the steps and flooded the landing be-

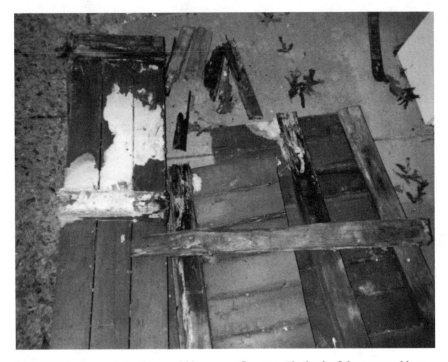

FIGURE 9.1. Decayed three-year-old basement flooring. The back of the removed basement flooring was covered with mold growth. The white material is a mass of hyphae called the mycelium, which is the mold's root structure digesting the wood. Some of the wood was so rotted that it crumbled. Photo by Steve Goselin; used with permission.

low. The threshold of the sliding door was at the same level as the patio, and water simply flowed into the bedroom, soaking the carpet. In another garden unit, roof water from two properties collected in a narrow alley between them and soaked into the old brick foundation walls. From there it ran along a concrete floor beneath the carpet, soaking the jute pad, carpet, and carpet dust.

Another woman became an independent consultant and worked from her home. The family expanded office space on the first floor and moved the living room down into a lavishly renovated space in the basement. Three years later, after living and working in her home nearly twenty-four hours a day, seven days a week, the woman developed terrible itchy rashes that were driving her crazy.

When I arrived, the first thing she did was point out some stains in the basement carpet. I did not expect them, because she had described how the carpet was laid on a plank subfloor raised above the concrete. I checked the stains with my moisture meter, and indeed they were wet. At first I was suspicious of the family dog, but the regularity of the pattern suggested the moisture had another cause.

I recommended she have a contractor lift some of the carpet and subfloor to determine the source. After creating asbestos-level dust containment conditions in the basement, the contractor found water on the concrete and extensive fungal growth on the back of the plank subfloor. Apparently rainwater had been leaking through cracks in the foundation and pooling on the masonry floor. Fungus had grown on the wood and between the planks, and moisture from the decaying wood had created the damp stain pattern.

The family ended up tearing out the entire floor, because the bottom of the subfloor was completely rotten beneath the carpeting. After the flooring was up, workers noticed decay in the wall structure, and they began to remove that. In the end the entire finished basement was demolished only three years after it had been created. The extent of this particular problem might have been discovered sooner had there been access to the wall structure. This is why I recommend leaving space between the walls and foundation in finished basements and installing an access panel so the area can be walked and inspected.

It's always risky to lay carpet directly on concrete, whether in a basement or on the first floor of a home built on a slab, since moisture condenses on the slab whenever the surface temperature is below the dew point. I prefer to see resilient or ceramic tile on the floors of finished basement rooms, but if homeowners insist on basement carpeting, I generally recommend laying it over a plywood subfloor resting on treated wood sleepers. Foam sheet insulation should be installed between the sleepers, with a vapor barrier above the sleepers but below the plywood subfloor. Unless sources of basement water are eliminated, however, there could still be fungal growth in the wood. (In addition, if the floor temperature is below the dew point, mold will grow in carpet dust.)

One couple I worked with bought a house with a long history of basement water problems. The seller had installed a sump pump and a drainage system under the floor to prevent basement flooding, but mold had already gotten a foothold. After living in their home for about three years, the new owners decided to spruce up the finished basement. They both worked many hours on the project, removing old carpeting and installing new vinyl flooring. They also moved their bedroom to a first-floor room adjacent to the basement stairway. They kept the door to the basement open because their children watched TV and played with their dog in the refurbished lower-level family room.

The wife began getting rashes on her face soon after the renovation was complete. At times her tongue swelled and her throat constricted. When I visited the home I was impressed by the glistening new floor in the basement room. It was clear they had worked very hard on the project. I was less impressed by the film of mildew on the lower two feet of all the paneled walls and the *Aspergillus* flourishing on many of the cellulose ceiling tiles.

The husband arrived after I had finished inspecting the basement and taking samples, and I felt it was important to explain to him directly all the problems I had observed. He and I (I was wearing an N95 NIOSH mask) walked through the basement for about ten minutes. At first he was quiet and avoided looking at me directly. The paneling was dark and the mildew layer was not readily visible, so as I went around I shone a bright flashlight obliquely across the surface, whereupon the colonies became quite obvious. I also pointed out white tufts of fungal growth (mycelium) protruding from the decorative ceiling beams. Little by little he became convinced as he recognized the extent of the contamination.

After our basement circumnavigation, I turned to tell him what I thought should be done to clean the basement. I noticed that as he spoke his voice had grown hoarse and mucus was dripping down his upper lip. When one member of a couple suffers from allergy symptoms, the other is often skeptical. Although he too had been experiencing symptoms when he went into his basement, he had remained in denial.

Although I did not suggest removing the beautiful new flooring, which was preferable to wall-to-wall carpeting, my extensive list of recommendations included removing all the ceiling and wall materials, including all partitions and nonstructural wood. I suggested they expose the ceiling structure and clean dust from joists, wires, and pipes with a HEPA vacuum. Spray painting the structure would help contain residual dust. The foundation walls could then be washed to eliminate loose material and coated with Thoroseal or painted.

The tile as well as the masonry floor in the mechanical room could also then be cleaned. I was very clear that this cleaning should be undertaken with asbestos-level containment measures to avoid contaminating habitable spaces with moldy dust. Last, I suggested operating a dehumidifier and keeping the basement door shut. Until the mitigation was complete, I encouraged the family to stay out of the basement (and keep the dog out too, for it could carry mold spores upstairs on its fur) and to keep the basement door tightly closed. After the basement was cleaned, I recommended eliminating all dust from the rest of the house with a HEPA vacuum.

Drowning at Home

Why do basements flood? Over the lifetime of every house, a flood will probably occur once or twice. External causes include a high water table, improper grading, and natural disasters such as torrential rains or river flooding. Some of the more common internal sources of basement flooding are broken water heaters, frozen pipes that burst, and broken washing machine hoses. If your finished basement floods, immediately remove the wet carpeting and padding as well as any damp upholstered furniture, because it is impossible to dry these items in place before mold and bacteria start to grow. You may be able to save the carpeting by having it professionally cleaned, but cushioned furniture and carpet padding, once soaked, should go on the trash heap.

After you have cleaned up the obvious basement water, don't forget about the most important potential source of home contamination: the bottom of your forced hot-air furnace or basement air conditioning system. I cannot tell you how many blower cabinets I have looked into that were full of mold from water on the basement floor. In one such home a young boy who had almost died from a bee sting was found in subsequent skin-prick testing to be sensitized to over thirty allergens, most probably including some of the fungi growing in the bottom of his family's neglected blower cabinet. In another home with a finished basement that had floor water and dampness owing to poor drainage, my footsteps squished on the carpet, leaving shoe-shaped puddles as I walked. Fiberglass insulation in the walls was still wet weeks after the last heavy rain. To a height of about three feet, the back of the basement drywall was black with *Stachybotrys* mold that was crawling with mites. I even found

Stachybotrys spores blowing out of the hot-air register on the first floor. Stains on the paper frame of the fiberglass furnace filter suggested that it too had been partially under water.

Sadly, the return air for the heating system came from the moldy basement family room. Both the parents and the children suffered from asthma as well as chronic sinus and respiratory problems. The mother was so ill and frustrated that she was prepared to tear the house down; they were even concerned about using the same foundation. They had the basement cleaned, but they also moved to a new house.

During catastrophic floods, government agencies, the Red Cross, and trained professionals step in to help the displaced. When you are the victim of a basement flood caused by a failed water heater or washer hose, the health consequences may also be dire, but often your only advice may come from a contractor.

CONDENSATION

Moisture can condense on masonry walls as well as floors, since these are always cooler than room air. One broker felt very lucky to list a lovely garden-level studio apartment. The unit had more light than one would expect from a basement unit. In one end wall, sliding glass doors opened to an inviting private patio. The apartment floors were flagstone, and the owner had plants hung everywhere, inside and out. The ambience was very appealing.

When the broker walked around the unit, she noticed that the edges of the floor along the walls were damp. She looked closely at the walls, which had been left in their original "fieldstone" condition, and saw a sheen of moisture all along the surface. The only way to prevent this situation is to either dehumidify or air condition the unit to minimize moisture buildup. In both cases the windows would have to be kept closed.

One of my clients neglected to take these precautions. To surprise his wife, he built a basement studio for her craft business. The room had shelves for storage and counters for work space, and she spent many productive hours there. Unfortunately the room was not adequately dehumidified or heated, and mildew grew on all the walls. She probably developed her sinus condition from exposure to the many spores in the air (one study found that over 90

percent of sinus infections involve fungi). I recommended the couple eliminate the room.

The likelihood of condensation is high in a small, cool space, particularly
if at least one wall is masonry. One woman had a chronic cough, and when I
visited the home I found wall-to-wall closets in a finished basement room. The
back wall of every closet was the masonry foundation. Moisture was condensing on the wall, and mold was spreading to the goods stored in the closet.
I suspected the woman coughed whenever she wore contaminated clothing.

Another condensation problem led to legal action. I was asked to help defend a siding installer being sued by a customer who claimed the vinyl siding
was responsible for the health problems he and his daughter were experiencing. According to the owner, the contractor had removed all the wood siding
on the house, exposing the wood plank sheathing to the weather. Before new
vinyl siding could be installed, heavy rains soaked the sheathing. The customer claimed the insulation in the wall cavities had also gotten wet. He believed the contractor had covered the walls with vinyl siding before they had
a chance to dry out. Within a month after the installation, the man's daughter
had to move out of her basement bedroom because of asthma symptoms, and
he himself began to experience more asthma symptoms and hoarseness.
Within a few months he was barely able to speak and was fired from his job,
which required a clear, audible voice. In addition to his health complaints, he
stated that the contractor had done a poor job installing the siding.

When I read the man's deposition I felt very sympathetic, and I wondered
if I would be able to support the contractor's position. When we arrived at
the house, though, I thought perhaps it was the wrong property, because I
could see none of the defects in the siding installation that the owner claimed
were present. As I entered, I also noticed that his housekeeping was less than
ideal. Cat food had been spilled in the kitchen, all the interior walls were
yellow with nicotine stains, and there were piles of clothing and other possessions on the floors. The porch had water-stained unfinished drywall on the
inside. Once thick but now flattened shag carpeting covered all the floors. I
started to have my doubts about the strength of his position.

I noticed that the door to the basement was open to give the family cat access to its basement litter box. As I descended the stairs I began to note the

odor of cat excrement. At the other end of the basement, I saw pawprints all along a sewer pipe that went from the basement into the dirt crawl space. The cat had shunned the litter box in favor of wider horizons. In addition, the basement was damp and all the walls and ceilings were covered with mildew. I removed the cover from the blower cabinet of the antique furnace and took samples of the dust. I later found that this too was contaminated with growing mold.

After my visit I seriously questioned that anything the installer could have done had caused the contamination I observed. It's possible that the nailing on the walls disturbed irritants already lurking inside the wall cavities, but it's doubtful that the single exposure of the building exterior to water could have produced the wretched indoor conditions I found. Only years of excessive humidity, condensation, and neglect could have created the "decor" in this partially finished basement.

INSULATION

I recommend using foil-covered sheet foam insulation on the foundation walls rather than fiberglass batts between the studs, for two reasons. First, if a basement floods, fiberglass absorbs the water and can retain the moisture for months. The wooden framing and the back of the drywall can get damp, and mold can proliferate. Solving this problem requires removing the wet insulation and replacing the lower portion of the drywall. Second, when fiberglass insulation is placed between the studs of the wood framing, a cold space is left between the back side of the finished wall and the interior side of the foundation wall. Moisture can condense in this space, encouraging fungal growth on dust and on the wood framing. Sheet foam insulation is placed flush against the foundation wall. The side of the insulation facing inward will be near the temperature of the heated, finished room (assuming no second layer of fiberglass insulation is placed up against the studs), so condensation will be at a minimum. In addition, sheet foam insulation does not absorb much moisture if there is a basement flood, and the area between the finished wall and the foundation wall will dry out faster.

One word of caution: the foam insulation should not rise to the top of the foundation wall. An inch or two of the concrete should be left visible for termite inspection. No debris should be left between the finished wall and the foundation wall.

HEATING FINISHED BASEMENTS

Many homeowners know how important it is to dehumidify finished basement rooms, but few realize it is vital to keep these rooms warm, not only when they are in use but throughout the colder months.

The joint where the masonry floor and wall meet is always the coolest part of a basement room, both because cold air sinks and because any object near a colder surface loses heat to that surface through radiation. The opposite occurs if you stand near a fireplace. The side of your body facing the fire feels warm because your body is cooler than the flame and thus absorbs some of the heat. If you were to stand in front of a block of ice, the opposite would occur: heat would radiate from your body and be absorbed by the ice. If two cold surfaces meet (such as the masonry floor and wall), the heat loss from an object near those surfaces is greater. An object in the corner where two walls meet the floor will lose more heat than if it is next to only one wall and will thus become even colder. For this reason temperatures at the outside corners of the foundation wall are usually the lowest, and the relative humidity is the highest. In a finished basement, insulated walls are cooled by heat loss from the walls' "exterior" sides to the cooler foundation (except where foam sheet insulation is placed against the foundation wall).

Think of the space where the wall meets the floor as the "joint zone." Within that colder area there is higher relative humidity and thus an increased chance of insect life and mildew. If carpet with nutrient dust is present, these conditions are conducive to almost year-round mildew growth and insect activity. If you look around a carpeted basement room, you will usually see most of the spiderwebs in the joint zone.

If you want to have carpet in a basement room, I recommend either using area rugs or bordering a larger carpet with up to eighteen inches of resilient or ceramic tile. With a smooth surface in the joint zone you can wipe up any moisture that may condense and eliminate settled dust more easily.

Heat sources (heat registers, baseboard convectors) are more difficult to keep clean than tiled surfaces, so heat sources placed in a joint zone can become homes for biological growth. In two split-level homes with carpeted, finished below-grade rooms, I removed dust samples from the bottoms of the clogged fin tubing of the baseboard heaters and in both cases found that the dust consisted of almost 30 percent *Aspergillus, Penicillium,* and *Cladosporium* mold growth. One owner had a chronic cough; the other also had respiratory distress. In both cases elevated levels of spores were found in the air in the finished lower levels. In another house, where the owner was sensitized to molds and suffered from chronic fatigue syndrome, I found *Penicillium* mold growing in the dust on a hot-air register in the joint zone of a basement room.

To avoid mold growth on heat sources, the emitters must be kept free of *all* dust. In addition, basement rooms must be dehumidified in the summer and heated consistently throughout the colder months. In a finished basement, the winter temperature should be the same as the temperature in your upstairs rooms, but not less than 65°F, and the relative humidity should be below 50 percent all year round.

PEST ODORS

In one single-family split-level house, the owners were concerned about a moldlike odor in the carpeted family room on the lower level. Because the house was built into a slope, the front wall of the lower-level room was partially below grade, but the rear was walk-out to grade (at ground level). The wife was a tutor and spent hours in the room each day, working with her students. Both she and her husband were worried that the odor might impair her livelihood as well as their health. They had already gone to considerable expense to replace the boiler and install a chimney liner in the mechanical room adjacent to the family room, in the mistaken notion that these steps would remove the odor.

I found that someone had installed a concrete patio at the rear exterior wall, completely covering the untreated wooden sill. Untreated wood should never be buried in concrete, because excess moisture from the ground will always lead to fungal decay (and to insects and other pests). In this case I could see a piece of the decayed sill at the lowest edge of the siding where some shingle was missing. The sill had been gnawed, probably by a rodent nesting there. I was never able to locate the exact source of the odor, but the carpenter who repaired the sill found that a rodent had chewed through the softened wood and gotten into the contiguous interior wall between the bathroom and the family room. The couple practically had to abandon the house while the fiberglass insulation from the rodent's nest was removed. Once the tufts of urine-soaked, moldy fiberglass were gone and the wall was repaired, the odor disappeared.

FINISHED PLAY SPACES

When children sit on contaminated furniture or play on moldy basement carpets, they disturb the irritating dust and not only breathe it in but carry it on their clothing to other parts of the house. I have looked at many homes where children had trouble breathing when they were playing on basement carpets full of mold and mites.

In one home, a friend of the owner's daughter experienced asthma symptoms as soon as she entered the house. The culprit was a couch in a finished basement, which contained more than 200 micrograms per gram of dust mite allergens. (More than 10 micrograms per gram is considered a risk for asthma, and this was one of the highest test results I have ever obtained.) When the couch was used, which was frequently, particulates rose from the cushions and even went up into the rest of the house with airflow through the open basement door.

Other pieces of furniture can also cause problems in basement play spaces, because surfaces close to the foundation wall tend to acquire mildew. In one finished basement room, I was surprised to see mildew growing at the front of a bookshelf rather than at the back, which was facing the exterior wall. I asked the owner, who had children with asthma, whether the bookshelf had ever been stored in another basement space. She told me that in her old house she had stored the shelf empty, pushed up against the foundation wall with the open shelves facing the masonry. In another ranch-style home with a below-grade family room, in addition to mold on the bookshelves, I found two children with asthma watching *Sesame Street* on a television set covered with *Aspergillus* mildew.

If your child has asthma or allergies, I cannot urge strongly enough that in a basement you avoid creating finished spaces in general and play spaces in particular.

A RESOUNDING NO!

If I could, I would encourage most homeowners to have finished basement rooms professionally dismantled. I would give a resounding no to adding finished rooms to a basement. I would tell tenants with allergies or asthma to move out of basement apartments.

If you have a finished basement, however, I hope the suggestions in this chapter will help you minimize potential contamination. Here are a few extra tips: divide the basement into as few rooms as possible; avoid small storage areas such as closets and built-in hinged-seat benches; and use louvered doors on closets. I don't recommend trying to heat finished basements with forced hot air, because it never seems to be warm enough at the floor. Use forced hot-water baseboard convectors (zoned separately from the rest of the house) or supplementary electric baseboard heaters.

Leave at least three inches between furniture and finished walls. If you are planning to have a couch in a finished basement room, use one covered with vinyl or leather, which acts as a barrier to prevent dust from settling into the cushioning or stuffing below. Whatever the material inside, if the surface fabric is permeable to dust, nutrients will accumulate within and moisture can penetrate, creating an environment conducive to biological growth. A futon is better than an overstuffed couch, because the mattress can be encased in an allergen-control covering, which provides the best protection against dust mites. Be cautious about manufacturers who claim their cushions will prevent mite colonization and mold growth. Nature is a powerful force; if food and water are accessible life will prevail, even if it is microscopic.

RECOMMENDATIONS

CARPETS

- Don't use carpeting in a basement space. If you insist on having carpet, lay it on a raised plywood subfloor rather than directly on the concrete, and install resilient vinyl or ceramic tile in the "joint zone."

- Area rugs are preferable to wall-to-wall carpeting, but it's best to lay them on tile or linoleum rather than directly on the concrete. Area rugs that rest on concrete must be periodically cleaned or thrown away.
- Basement carpets or rugs that have gotten wet even once should be discarded if they smell or cannot be dried out within hours or if the water contained sewage.
- If possible, have flooded rugs and carpets professionally cleaned and dried off-site.

CONDITIONING AND HEATING THE AIR

- Dehumidify below-grade spaces and maintain the relative humidity below 50 percent.
- Heat a finished basement consistently throughout the colder months. Keep the baseboard convectors and registers free of all dust.
- Baseboard heat is better than hot-air heat for all spaces, but particularly for basements.

ODORS

- If there are animal odors in the basement, you may have to remove soiled building materials.

USES

- Don't let children play in moldy basements, whether the spaces are finished or unfinished. Adults too should avoid spending prolonged time there.
- If you have allergies or asthma, don't exercise or live in a below-grade space. In addition, avoid houses with finished basements.
- If you are retired, don't spend long periods in a moldy basement.

MISCELLANEOUS

- When finishing a basement, use sheet foam insulation against the foundation wall rather than fiberglass insulation between the wall studs. (Unfortunately, this cannot be done with an uneven stone foundation.)
- If your basement is moldy, have it cleaned professionally using containment measures to avoid spreading the dust throughout the house. If there is a mildew odor, even if you smell it only intermittently, the basement is moldy.

10

Heating and Cooling with Air

This chapter covers furnaces, heat pumps, and central air conditioning. Chapter 11 continues the discussion of heating with a look at electric baseboard heat, boilers, and problems associated with fuel.

HOT-AIR HEATING SYSTEMS

Today most new homes in America are built with central hot-air heating systems. Such a system uses a network of ducts to distribute air from a heat source. Years ago, before the advent of central heat, separate rooms were heated by fireplaces or stoves. When people began to think about how a single heat source might warm the entire house, two questions no doubt arose: where to put the "fire," and how to distribute the heat from the fire to the other rooms.

In the first central hot-air systems, a basement heat source warmed air. The heat source was placed in the basement, and the air it warmed rose by convection through ducts and registers to the rooms above. Such a furnace consisted of a cast-iron stove mostly surrounded by a sheet-metal case into which the ducts were inserted. The front doors of the coal stove were not encased in the sheet metal, so coal could be shoveled in and ashes removed and so air could flow into the stove to fuel combustion. Combustion gases were eliminated through a metal vent pipe that ran from the stove into a chimney. There was a large opening at the bottom of the sheet-metal case to let basement air into the space between the stove and the case. The cast-iron walls of the coal

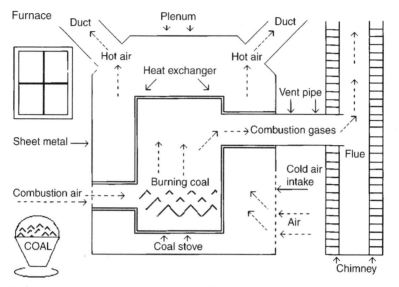

The furnace consists of a coal stove surrounded by a sheet metal enclosure. There are two separate air pathways. Combustion air for burning the coal enters at the lower left. Combustion gases from burning coal exit the heat exchanger at the upper right, enter the vent pipe, and flow into the chimney flue. Air for heating the house enters at the cold air intake, flows around the heat exchanger, and rises into the plenum and ducts.

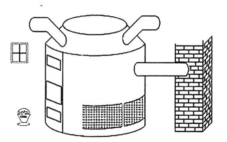

FIGURE 10.1. Schematic drawing of a gravity hot-air furnace (side view). This diagram illustrates the two separate airflows that take place in a gravity hot-air heating system.

stove transferred heat to this air, which then rose through the ducts and warmed the house. The stove walls were thus the first "heat exchangers" in hot-air systems. (The walls also prevented toxic combustion gases produced by the burning coal from mixing with the warm air between the heat exchanger and the sheet-metal case.) These early furnaces were called gravity hot-air systems, because gravity is what causes colder, denser air to sink and warmer, less dense air to rise.

To carry warm air only by convection, the ducts in a gravity system had to be quite large—at least eight to ten inches in diameter. If you have ever seen these older systems, you know the large ducts take up quite a bit of room in the basement. Because these early furnace units were so big and had many ducts extending outward at the top, some people called them octopuses.

These octopuses depended on a constant source of cold air infiltration (flow in) into the basement and on very leaky windows, doors, and attics for exfiltration (flow out). Think of the heating pattern as a cycle of air. Hot air rises, so as a furnace of this type heated the basement air, which then rose into the ducts, air pressure in the basement dropped. Outside air was then pushed into the basement through leaks in foundations and basement windows and doors to replace the air flowing upward in the ducts. The heated air rising by convection leaked out of the house through similar openings in upstairs walls and in the attic.

Gravity hot-air heating systems were inefficient. First, because they heated only very cold basement or outside air, they required a lot of fuel (coal was cheap back then). Second, because the warmed air was leaking out of the house, no heated air circulated within a home more than once. Third, the systems had to be designed very carefully, for all the ducts had to have the proper slope to maintain the convection cycle. Warm air would not flow into a duct with a downward turn, and any room fed by an incorrectly pitched duct would remain cold.

A blower and return duct were later added to increase the efficiency and comfort of a central hot-air heating system. Instead of depending on convection to move the air, a forced hot-air system uses a mechanical fan or blower to circulate the air at a rate of between 800 and 1,500 cubic feet per minute. Much larger volumes of warm air could now be moved through smaller ducts. In addition, the slope of the duct was no longer relevant, because the air was being forced through the system. This means that ducts could go up, over, and around obstacles. (Today flexible plastic ducts are used in forced hot-air systems.) The return duct offers an avenue for air to enter the system from inside rather than outside the house. Air that has already been heated thus returns to the furnace and is recirculated, so less energy is required to maintain a consistent interior temperature.

When blowers were first introduced, furnace designers feared the increased airflow would pull debris such as paper and dust into the system, where it might be ignited. To prevent this, a coarse filter was added to the intake. Other improvements included designing furnaces that could burn oil or gas, not just coal, allowing for smaller heat exchangers that could still produce intense heat. Electric furnaces, which burn no fuel, were also introduced. In an electric furnace, air is blown over red-hot coils very similar to those in a toaster.

A further development was the heat pump, which consists of a split system: an indoor unit and an outdoor unit. The blower and heat exchange coil (together called an air handling unit, or AHU) are indoors and the compressor is outdoors. Through heat exchange with the outside air, a heat pump system can both heat and cool inside air. Most heat pumps also have electric heating coils, called emergency heat, to act as backup if the compressor breaks down.

A Closed System

In all homes, air leaks in and out (mostly at gaps around windows and doors) owing to pressure differences between the air inside and outside the house. The rate at which air is replaced in a building is called the *air exchange* or *ventilation rate,* and it is measured in "air changes per hour" (ACH). In a typical poorly insulated, leaky Victorian-era house, all the interior air may be replaced by outdoor air each hour (1 ACH). Heat bills are high in Victorians because nearly every hour a volume of air equal to that of the entire interior space of the house has to be heated from outside temperature to indoor temperature.

In a modern, more "tightly" constructed and better insulated home, the air exchange rate is reduced to about 0.25 ACH or less. Because newer homes have lower air exchanges, the heating systems recirculate the inside air. This may save money, but it also increases exposure to all kinds of pollutants, including combustion gases, radon, and formaldehyde, as well as by-products of biological growth. For example, if there is mold growth in the furnace blower cabinet and the ducts in a newer home, less fresh air is available to dilute the mold spores and odors. The effects can range from occasional sneezing, coughing, and headaches to year-round allergy symptoms, respiratory distress, or even disabling physical pain.

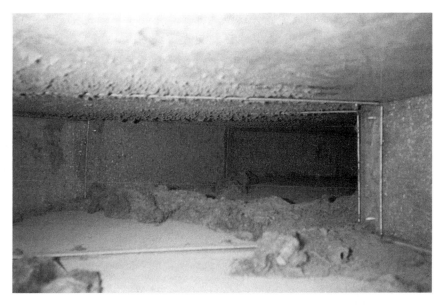

FIGURE 10.2. Inside of a dirty heating duct. The pile of dust at the bottom of this duct is typical of returns in forced hot-air systems. The dust consists mostly of human skin scales. Paper and cloth fibers help to keep the mass intact. Numerous insects forage in the dust for nutrients. In moist areas, mold also feeds on the dust. Photo by Rick Hughes; used with permission.

HEATING DUCTS

A woman with asthma called me because she suspected the mold odor in her kitchen was causing her headaches. In the floor were both a hot-air supply register and a return grille (a register has dampers for airflow adjustment; a grille does not). The grille sucked kitchen air into the hot-air heating system, and the duct passed through a damp, cold crawl space under the kitchen. The woman had already had her ducts cleaned, but the company forgot to include the kitchen return duct, which was clogged with hair and a variety of materials ripe for biological growth, such as crumbs and skin scales. I tested the airflow at the duct with a smoke pencil and found that with the heating system turned off, air moved into the room by convection from the duct. Before I left the house I used a mirror and a flashlight to show her the festering mat that had been accumulating within the duct beneath her return grille.

Back at the office, I looked with a microscope at a sample of the dust from the return duct and found it consisted of about 30 percent mold that was flourishing on the food and other biodegradable materials. Numerous dust mites and other insects were enjoying the moldy banquet. When the dust was disturbed, these irritants became airborne.

The owner was so horrified at the appearance of the leftover dust in the return that as soon as I left she had the duct cleaning company come back to remove the debris. The cleaners did not exercise the careful mitigation efforts required around a person who has asthma, however, so even more irritants were released into the air. It's not surprising that the woman's breathing got much worse. *Utmost care must be exercised in removing contaminants from the environment of a person who is sensitized.* In fact, sensitized individuals should insist that the duct cleaning company do a site evaluation before undertaking the job, to determine the scope of the work and to explain its services in detail.

In another home, a woman and her son were both miserable owing to mold odors and allergens coming out of contaminated ductwork that passed through a cold, damp crawl space. The problem was so severe that though she had purchased her home only three months before, she was looking for another place to live. I was amazed to learn that she had paid for a home inspection before she bought the house and that the inspector had never even mentioned the crawl space or the moldy debris sitting in the ducts beneath the registers.

The owner had chosen this inspector from a very short list given to her by the real estate agent. Rather than selecting a home inspector from a real estate agent's list, buyers should obtain a referral from a friend or an attorney. A real estate agent, after all, in most cases is representing the seller. I also recommend that buyers use an inspector who is a member of the American Society of Home Inspectors (ASHI), which provides a code of ethics and standards of practice and requires testing and education for membership. In this case, had the home inspector discussed the problems associated with heat ducts running through crawl spaces, the woman might not have purchased the home, since both she and her son had serious allergies.

Fungus (mold) readily grows in damp cavities, particularly if the spaces are close to masonry. A duct in a concrete slab is just such a place. In the home of a family with allergies, no ducts should pass through a slab, since it is virtually certain the accumulated dust will become contaminated. In addition, if the soil beneath your home has been treated for termites and your ducts pass through or beneath a concrete slab, pesticide may evaporate through gaps in metal ducts or through the walls of porous ducts and contaminate the air that flows through them.

Wherever they are, dirty ducts can impair health. In one case I investigated, a woman had been experiencing debilitating symptoms including migraines, muscle pains, swelling in the backs of her knees and calves, and tenderness in her wrists. She left her house for the first time in several years to go on a week's vacation. While she was away all her symptoms gradually disappeared, and she was elated. She was able to move without pain for the first time in three years. Within hours after she came home, however, all her symptoms returned. Her doctor recommended she call me, because he suspected an environmental trigger in her house was responsible.

I generally take Burkard air samples to determine the level of mold spores and try to identify the mold genus. When my clients are experiencing severe symptoms, however, I sometimes take Andersen air samples and send the petri dishes to a mycologist to determine what species of mold are present. In this case the laboratory found elevated levels of several kinds of mold, including *Aspergillus ochraceus,* a species that produces a mycotoxin called ochratoxin-A. This very dangerous mycotoxin can suppress the immune system and disrupt kidney function. Some studies have even found it to be carcinogenic.

Aspergillus often grows on grains, and because this mycotoxin is so poisonous, animal feeds are routinely tested for it. Such testing is rarely undertaken in indoor air quality investigations, however. My client wanted to take this extra step, so more duct dust samples were gathered by a duct cleaning company and sent to a specialized laboratory. In one sample the lab found a concentration of over 1,500 parts per billion (ppb) of ochratoxin-A (typically, grains are considered contaminated if there are even a few ppb of ochratoxin-A). A lab scientist told me this was the highest level he had ever seen in any sample of any type, and he recommended the woman immediately move out. Her symptoms disappeared as soon as she stopped living in the house.

But there is more to this story. The woman had been there for over twenty years. Why had she developed these problems only in the past three years? Three events had occurred that might have contributed to the extraordinary mold growth and its distribution. First, a water heater on the first floor had burst, possibly sending water into the ducts. Second, she had insulation installed around the ducts, and the installation had disturbed the dust in the ducts. And third, she had added a furnace humidifier that was elevating the moisture levels in the system. In addition, two other conditions had existed for a long time. First, she had never had the ducts or furnace cleaned since moving into the house. Second, the ducts passed through an unconditioned crawl space with less than two feet of clearance between the floor structure and the soil. At some locations the rusted-out ducts were resting in the dirt.

This story is still unfolding and there is more research to be done, but it was clear that her exposure to the air in her home was making her very ill. I did not recommend the house be *razed,* but I did recommend it be *raised* to create headroom for a proper basement (eliminating the crawl space). I did not recommend cleaning the furnace and the ducts, since they were so deteriorated and contaminated. Instead I encouraged the owner to eliminate the furnace and ducts (with asbestos-level mitigation procedures) and replace them with a hot-water heating system.

Should People Clean Their Ducts?

Studies do not generally support duct cleaners' claim that the process will reduce dust and allergens in the house, but I believe this is because, more often than not, duct cleaning is done improperly and inadequately.

Let's step back a moment. I feel very strongly that people with allergies and asthma should not live in homes with forced hot-air heating. There is just too great a chance for circulation of contaminants. Some of my prepurchase home inspection clients have even replaced hot-air systems before moving in. If you have such a system, however, it's extremely important to keep the interior of the ducts and the furnace free of dust and debris. With proper filtration, ducts should not have to be cleaned more than once every five or ten years.

Do not clean ducts on your own. (If you use a leaky vacuum cleaner, for example, you could spread mold and mycotoxin into the house air.) Instead, hire a company that uses brushes and HEPA vacuums to clean. Using a truck-mounted vacuum and an air "whip" in place of a brush to loosen dust just

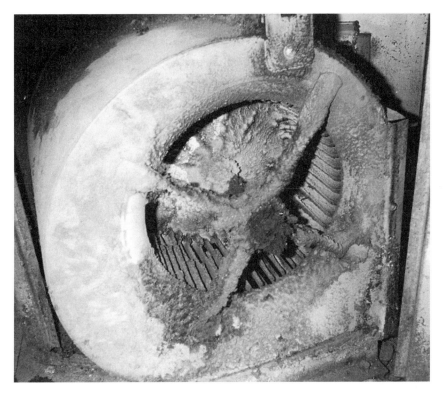

FIGURE 10.3. A dirty blower in a furnace. This blower is coated with dust. The pattern of the dark staining suggested long-term exposure to dripping water. Such dust is certain to contain growing microorganisms such as mold or bacteria. Soiled mechanical equipment like this should never be in the flow of conditioned air that people breathe. Photo by Rick Hughes; used with permission.

isn't adequate. To reach the ends of ducts, every floor, wall, and ceiling register must be removed during cleaning. In the basement, a hole may be cut into a duct where access through existing openings is limited. Making holes in the duct does not damage the system as long as the hole is properly sealed after the job is completed. If anyone in your family is sensitized to the dust, great caution should be used during cleaning. The ducts should be under negative pressure so that any dust made airborne within the system is not released into the house air, and whenever possible, duct surfaces should be HEPA vacuumed by physical contact with the vacuum tool. People with allergies should vacate the house while the ducts are being cleaned.

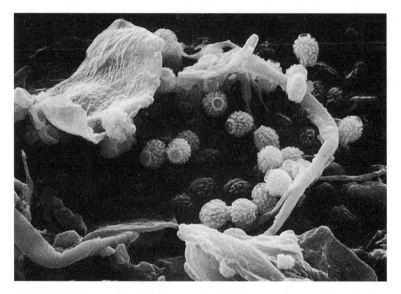

FIGURE 10.4. *Aspergillus* mold growing in the dust on a furnace blower. These *Aspergillus* spores and hyphae were present in a fine layer of dust, barely visible on the blades of a six-year-old furnace. (In the upper left and lower right corners are two light-colored skin scales.) Spores from the blower were dispersed into airflow from the heating system, and the family was suffering from allergies. (2,000× SEM)

Most people think it is adequate to clean only the ducts (thus "duct cleaning"), but unfortunately there is far more to an air conveyance system. It's essential that the blower and blower cabinet as well as the air conditioning coil (if present) be cleaned at the same time and with the same caution. Whenever possible, the blower should be removed for cleaning. After a system is cleaned, there should be little or no dust visible in the entire heating system. (Tell the service provider you plan to check with a mirror and a flashlight.) This is particularly important for an allergy-prone family. One woman from out of state called me because her father, who had asthma, was hospitalized with a collapsed lung after his ducts had been inadequately and sloppily cleaned.

I have been contacted by many families suffering from allergies even after they had their ducts cleaned. In one case an ultraviolet "disinfectant system" had been installed, and in other cases electronic filters had been added to the furnace. None of these costly "solutions" worked, because the blowers and blower cabinets were untouched and thus were left contaminated with mold.

Some cleaning companies advertise various duct treatments such as spray coatings and biocides. I do not believe these are needed, except during cleaning of the air conditioning coil and condensate tray. Spray coatings will glue the residual dust in place and only make it harder to clean the ducts in the future. Biocides may kill some percentage of the organisms present in the duct, but just because mold and bacteria are killed doesn't mean they won't still be irritating if they become aerosolized. In addition, as soon as the solution dries out and a new layer of dust containing new spores and bacteria accumulates, biological growth can recommence when moisture conditions are suitable. Finally, some biocides may become airborne on coated dust particles and cause air quality problems of their own.

There are two types of nonmetallic ducts that in my opinion cannot be cleaned adequately. One type, made from fiberglass board coated on the outside with aluminum foil, can be rectangular (called duct board) or round. In residential installations, when the interior fiberglass surface becomes soiled and contaminated, it cannot be cleaned because it is porous. Mold-contaminated fiberglass ducts should be replaced.

The other type of duct is flexible and consists of plastic on the inside and outside, with fiberglass in between and a metal spiral to stiffen the inner plastic and maintain the duct opening. The interior plastic surface is smooth, but the metal spiral creates ridges, making the duct difficult to clean. In addition, the duct is often squashed during installation because it is so flexible, and this makes it hard to reach all interior surfaces. Compared with most solid metal ducts, flexible ducts are inexpensive, and it is cheaper to replace them than to clean them if they are in an accessible space such as the attic. Unfortunately, flexible ductwork is sometimes installed in ceilings, where it cannot be replaced without great expense. This is why I recommend that installers use metal ducts (see chapter 13).

Flexible ducts are covered in about an inch of fiberglass insulation held in place by a vinyl wrap. The wrap on some flexible ducts spontaneously deteriorates (a condition I have seen primarily in attics), allowing the insulation to fall off. Once this happens you are heating or cooling your attic rather than your living spaces, and outside moisture will condense on the exposed hoses if they are cold. Periodically check the exterior of your flexible attic ducts and replace them as necessary.

Return Ducts

There are two sides to the forced hot-air cycle: the supply side and the return side. Usually there is a supply duct to every room in a home. Many years ago, when hot-air heat was first installed, there was also a return duct in every room. This balanced the airflow. Today contractors save money by installing only one or two returns, usually in central areas of the home: in the floor or ceiling of a common hallway, for example.

Because return ducts draw house air in, they tend to have the largest accumulations of dust and debris. (In addition, I have found toys, combs, leaves, and candies piled up inside return ducts.) If a return duct is close to the basement floor, which is generally cooler because of heat loss to the concrete, the high relative humidity there can lead to mold growth in the dust. Sometimes a return duct is placed within the concrete floor. This is not a good idea, since a return in the basement floor may draw in radon gas as well as moisture.

Return ducts usually are not in the concrete but in the basement ceiling, and they are connected to return grilles in the floor above. Occasionally I inspect a home in which the return grille on the first floor has been covered with a rug. This starves the furnace of air and limits the supply of warmer air into the rooms. In addition, the reduced pressure created in the air-starved ducts can bend the metal inward when the blower turns on. In such cases, when the blower shuts off the metal makes a popping noise as the ducts return to their original shape. If you hear a noise like this when your blower turns on or off, be sure a rug is not covering the grille. If your grille isn't blocked, hire a professional to investigate the cause, because the popping means that your return airflow is somehow restricted or inadequate.

Whether the system is starved for air or not, there will always be reduced pressure in the return duct. If there are gaps or leaks anywhere in the return system, unwanted air from wall cavities or the basement can enter, carrying contaminants with it. If a leaky return duct passes through a moldy crawl space, odors, spores, and moisture are circulated through the house.

A particularly leaky type of return uses a panned bay—a duct created by enclosing the space between two wood floor joists with sheet metal. The top of this duct consists of the subfloor, the sides consist of the floor joists, and the bottom is the sheet metal. Contractors use panned bays so they don't have to reduce the ceiling height in the basement with an additional duct. I often see big openings in panned bays to accommodate wires and pipes. In addition, more often than not these ducts are inadequately sealed at the top and the ends.

Sometimes the return is not even ducted but is on the furnace itself and consists only of an opening in the blower cabinet wall. In many jurisdictions this is not allowed because it is such a dangerous practice. For example, with a gas-fired furnace, the pressure reduction in the basement caused by the blower can cause downdrafting at the furnace chimney flue. This can introduce combustion gases into the supply air, and if carbon monoxide is present it can cause illness or death.

A return can be created accidentally at the furnace if the blower door is not fastened shut. I was asked to investigate just such a situation in which an entire family of four was hospitalized. In the middle of the night the door to the blower cabinet of the furnace had fallen off, and the next time the furnace turned on it drew over 1,000 cubic feet of air per minute from the basement, lowering the air pressure. Air then flowed from the chimney flue back into the basement, carrying combustion products that included carbon monoxide. The furnace then circulated the carbon monoxide throughout the house. I always recommend installing carbon monoxide detectors at or near the basement ceiling, because combustion gases are hot and therefore rise. Combustion gases can also enter your living spaces through a damaged chimney or a cracked or rusted heat exchanger, so it's sensible to have carbon monoxide detectors on every level of your home, but at least outside the bedrooms. In addition, always check that the blower cabinet door is securely in place. (New furnaces have an interlock switch at the blower door. If the door is not properly secured, the furnace will not operate.)

Even when return ducts are properly installed, the cabinet holding the blower is a part of the return system, because air is being drawn into that space. Now and then, in homes with ducted returns, I find blower cabinets without bottoms. Depending on the size of the floor gap, this improper installation may negate the purpose of the return duct and allow unfiltered air from the level of the basement floor to be drawn into the heating system. In several homes that had been flooded, owners didn't realize water had soaked into the open bottom of the blower cabinet and moistened thick mats of dust that had accumulated over the years. Mold and bacteria grew there and released allergens into the airflow. If your basement floods, don't forget to clean and disinfect the entire interior of the blower cabinet, including the bottom, whether there is sheet metal or not, for water could have seeped in. And be sure to replace the furnace filter.

Another common practice is to leave out the return duct when the furnace is in a mechanical closet on a level other than the basement. I usually find such arrangements in condominiums and town houses. In this situation there is usually a louvered door to let air in. In some installations, though, I have seen mechanical closets with openings left in the ceiling to furnish the return air. This air is often sucked through building cavities to the furnace. This is particularly foolish in very old homes, because dust from the cavities supplying the makeup air may contain years of accumulated allergens.

One allergic condominium owner had serious problems because her heat pump was installed in a mechanical closet without a ducted return. A hole was left in the wall so air could come from the unit's laundry room, but the laundry room had a solid door. There was also an opening in the ceiling of the laundry and the adjacent hallway. I suppose the designer thought air would flow from the ceiling grille in the hallway into the laundry room and from there into the mechanical closet.

This wasn't what happened, unfortunately. The mechanical closet on the owner's floor was wedged between those of the condominiums above and below. There were large openings—larger than needed—for pipes in the floors and ceilings, interconnecting the three closets. One of my client's complaints was that she could smell coffee in the morning before she wanted to get up, because the owner of the condominium below hers was an early riser. In the evening she was choked by cigarette smoke that got drawn into her mechanical closet from the unit above.

Perhaps she wouldn't have minded these smells so much if she hadn't also been experiencing year-round bronchitis, sore throat, and allergies. She was late meeting me at her home for my site visit because she was returning from the emergency room after a severe episode of breathing difficulty. Before moving into the condominium she had been an avid jogger, but she hadn't been able to run for months.

I found that the filter in the mechanical closet had fallen to the floor and the air conditioning coil was covered with mold. In addition, because of the shared airflow among the three units, any contamination in the other units was distributed throughout her unit too. I recommended she stop using the heat pump and put in baseboard electric heat instead. Because the wall-to-wall carpets contained dust from the moldy heat pump, I encouraged her to install hardwood flooring. I also told her to get rid of her down comforter and pillow.

Within days of turning off the heat pump, she was able to jog again. Once she installed wood flooring, all her symptoms decreased until one day when she returned home from errands and once again had such trouble breathing that she was hospitalized. She subsequently found out that the filters on heat pumps throughout the buildings had been changed that day. These heat pumps were also contaminated, and dust had become airborne in the hallways. In the end, because she could not control the air quality in the common areas of the building, she was forced to sell her condominium and move.

FURNACE FILTERS

Many people think the purpose of a furnace filter is to clean the house air. The typical fiberglass air filter (frequently sixteen by twenty inches by one inch thick) found in most hot-air systems was designed, as I noted earlier, to keep paper and other debris away from the heat exchanger, not to keep the house air clean. If you hold this type of filter up to the light you can see right through it. Such filters may stop feathers, but they will not stop many microscopic pollen or mold spores from being recirculated.

People with allergies or asthma sometimes change their furnace filters monthly in the mistaken notion that this will keep the air cleaner. You could replace a typical furnace filter every day and it would not improve the quality of the air in your house. In fact in one Canadian study researchers found that over the first few hours of use, fiberglass furnace filters, unlike all other filters tested, slightly increased the number of airborne particulates (probably because the filters were dusty when first installed). Although fiberglass furnace filters are widely used, *in my opinion they are virtually useless for ameliorating air quality.*

There are more efficient air filters, however, that do remove mold spores and pollen from the air. For example, a pleated media filter, which you can't see through, is available in many hardware stores. This filter has more surface area and finer holes and thus is more effective. I prefer such filters even though they are several times as expensive as fiberglass filters. But the blowers in some systems do not have adequate power to draw air across the better filters, so you should check with the manufacturer of your system.

Another even more efficient type of media filter can be installed in a forced hot-air system. This filter, ideal for allergy sufferers because it is approximately 40 percent efficient, is much larger (about twenty-five inches square by six inches thick) and requires a separate installation as well as a duct modification. When I take Burkard samples of the air coming from systems with this type of thick media filter, I find very few particulates.

This is not the case when I look at systems with loudly touted, expensive electronic filters. Although electronic filters can initially be more than 90 percent efficient, dust quickly accumulates on the high-voltage wires, and the filter's efficiency drops. Manufacturers usually recommend that electronic filters be cleaned four times a year, but even this is inadequate. I find these filters need cleaning at least once a month. Unfortunately, filters are often in relatively inaccessible basement or attic spaces that people are reluctant to enter. I find that in most homes the components of the electronic filters have never been cleaned, and there is consequently no filtration for the system at all other than the metal mesh prefilter that is usually present. If you are planning to upgrade the filtration on your system, I would not recommend an electronic filter. In addition, a humidifier should never be installed "upwind" of an electronic filter, because aerosolized particulates from the humidifier land on the filter and reduce its efficiency.

I also don't recommend washable electrostatic filters, not because they are inadequate but rather because I have never seen one that was ever cleaned. In addition, it's virtually impossible to remove all the dust, and repeatedly washing a dirty filter encourages biological growth. The best type of filter is one you throw away when it is soiled.

Typically the filter is positioned at the furnace just before the air enters the blower cabinet. If you are using an efficient media filter and there is some distance of return duct, I suggest also using an inexpensive fiberglass filter at the return grille to stop larger dust particles from entering the return duct system. Regardless of the type of filter you have, it should be replaced according to the manufacturer's recommendation. It should also be the right size, and the access to the filter should be covered; otherwise unfiltered air will enter the system. *Don't waste your money on any filter ("bypass") system, no matter how efficient it is, if it filters only part of the return air!*

FURNACE HUMIDIFIERS

Many people believe forced hot-air heat is dry, so they install humidifiers on the system. After you read this section, I hope you'll think twice about doing this.

A retired couple purchased a condominium in a three-year-old complex. They were the first family to occupy the unit. During the sell-out phase the unit had been used for storage, and it was the last condominium to be sold. As soon as the couple moved in, they had a contractor install a furnace humidifier. In addition, since the unit was air conditioned, they never opened their windows. Shortly thereafter the wife started having chronic upper-respiratory infections. Her husband sneezed frequently, and both had trouble sleeping. The wife was a smoker, but her physician thought her infections were made worse not by her smoking but by something in the house.

I entered the scene six months later. I measured the moisture content of the inside air and found it was four times that of the outside air. I went to the mechanical closet and saw a drum-type humidifier consisting of a cylinder-shaped sponge pad that rotated within a tray of water. When I removed the cover and the pan, I was overwhelmed by the putrid odor. Floating on the surface of the tray were numerous large colonies of mold. The water in the entire tray was colored amber and brown by filamentous growths beneath the surface, and there was also a thick layer of crystallized minerals. I looked at a sample of the water with a microscope and saw bacteria and several genera of fungi, including *Alternaria* and *Epicoccum*. Both of these are associated with allergies and respiratory distress.

I had also taken Burkard air samples in the condominium, and considering the extraordinary extent of contamination in the humidifier tray, I was surprised to find there were not many mold spores in the air. But even when I don't find high levels of particulates in the air, people may still experience increased asthma and allergy symptoms while they are in their homes. In such situations the humidifier tray may contain crystallized minerals along with biological growth and its by-products—the chemicals that mold and bacteria contain and excrete. When the water films break on the humidifier sponge and the water drips from the rotating drum, irritants may become airborne within small water droplets. When the water droplets evaporate, even smaller particulates remain suspended. If they become airborne, any dust particles from the tray water will also be covered with irritants. Any of these irritants can be inhaled. They settle on furniture and carpets and can be reaerosolized when the surfaces are disturbed.

In this case I found *Epicoccum* spores in dust from the carpet. In the blower cabinet I found a dried-out amber flake of minerals full of *Alternaria* spores. This flake was a clear indication that particulates were being ejected from the humidifier and entering airflows in the system.

Why was there such prolific mold growth in the humidifier tray? I hadn't a clue until I looked at the dust samples from the hall floor. These contained typ-

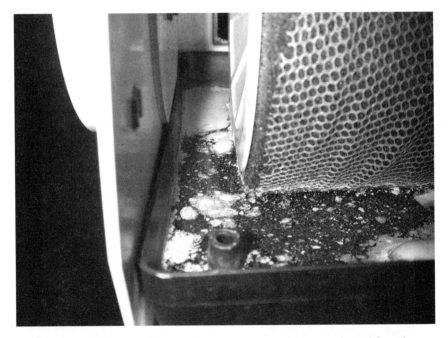

FIGURE 10.5. The evaporative pad and water reservoir of a furnace humidifier. The numerous small white dots floating on the water's surface are clusters of actinomycetes that produce spores the size of bacteria. Because they are so small, the spores can easily be dispersed and suspended in the furnace airflow.

ical settled air particulates (skin scales, cellulose), but what was most unusual was that almost half of the dust consisted of starch granules. I asked the owner if she used body powder containing starch or whether she did a lot of baking. She said no, but she told me that while her condo was being used for storage, contractors might have mixed starch-containing wallpaper paste in the unit for their work elsewhere. The starch granules from the dry powder must have become airborne and accumulated in the ducts. When the heating system was operating, granules found their way into the humidifier water, where they became nutrients for mold and bacteria. Ironically, another of the woman's complaints was that she had to constantly clean dust from the floor and other surfaces, and she had always wondered why there was so much.

Because the mold spores found in the carpeting most likely had originated in the humidifier, I recommended removing the carpeting. I also recommended removing the humidifier and having the ducts and furnace professionally cleaned. A few years later the woman called me. She was so congested that her voice was barely audible. She reported they had had the heating system cleaned and the humidifier removed, but that they had kept the contaminated carpeting. I told her I thought the carpeting was releasing airborne irritants every time someone walked across the fleecy surface.

One organization sponsored a study of humidifiers undertaken by university scientists. The study concluded that furnace humidifiers are not a source of bacteria. How is it, then, that I find a connection between contaminated furnace humidifiers and clients with symptoms? And why do these people usually feel better when the humidifiers are removed?

The study was conducted in a laboratory, using a model setup that consisted of a self-contained, sterile duct system with a HEPA filter and a humidifier. The water in the humidifier was initially sterile and contained no nutrients to support any microbial life. In the experiment, the researchers noted that many of the bacteria that were placed into the humidifier water died rapidly. The results of this study would have been very different had they used a humidifier and some ducts from one of my clients' heating systems.

During one of my indoor air quality lectures, I asked a group of seventy experienced home inspectors if any one of them had ever seen a furnace humidifier that was operating properly. This group represented over 100,000 completed home inspections. I didn't see a single hand go up, but I did hear a lot of laughter.

As you might guess, I would discourage anyone from using a furnace humidifier, except possibly the trickle or steam type, which have no water reservoirs to support biological growth. Any system with a humidifier should be inspected at least monthly, however, to be sure there are no leaks and no water is soaking into any fiberglass material that may be lining the furnace or ducts. In addition to creating a growth environment for contaminants, a leaking furnace humidifier can corrode a heat exchanger or a furnace vent pipe, allowing potentially lethal combustion gases to escape.

AIR CONDITIONING

Whether part of a hot-air heating system or a heat pump system, in my opinion *central air conditioning represents one of the greatest potential sources of biological contamination indoors.* As you may remember from chapter 3, in an air conditioning system air is blown across a cold coil. In apartments or condominiums, cold water may be circulated to the coil from a central chiller. In single-family homes, compressors may supply refrigerant. Regardless of the cooling source, as the air cools moisture condenses on the coil and water drops into a pan called a condensate tray. Dust and moisture meet in the tray and on the coil. The fiberglass lining can also become wet if water splashes onto it from either the coil, a leaking condensate tray, or a condensate tray with an improperly installed drain line. These conditions are ideal for biological growth. Even if parts of the moldy soup dry out, particulates can become aerosolized by airflows.

Heating, ventilating, and air conditioning (HVAC) technicians focus on keeping the equipment maintained so it will be efficient and will provide a comfortable level of cooling rather than concerning themselves with indoor air quality. The homeowner and the technician therefore should share the responsibility for maintaining the central air conditioning system, particularly in families with allergies or asthma. If you or anyone living in your house or apartment has allergies or asthma, be particularly vigilant about keeping your air conditioning system spotless.

One young woman rented a town house in which previous tenants and the landlord were not very careful about keeping the central air conditioning system clean. She moved in during the summer and within two weeks began to feel short of breath. A physician found that her blood oxygen was low. Several months later she was diagnosed with a peculiar pulmonary condition, eosinophilia granuloma. At the same time, she found out she was pregnant. Her doctors were greatly concerned that the fetus might have been affected by the oxygen deprivation she had experienced early in her pregnancy. She vacated the town house and her symptoms decreased, but they resumed whenever she returned to the unit to pick up possessions.

I found that the condensate tray for the air conditioning coil was leaking into the fiberglass lining below. The insulation was very dirty and full of mold. Airflows passed over the contaminated insulation, disturbing the irritants and carrying them into the air. Luckily for this young woman, her baby was born healthy.

In another air conditioning horror story, a man with a history of sinusitis moved into his new home and shortly afterward developed nosebleeds, swollen and teary eyes, and dizziness. I removed the cover that concealed the heat pump coil and was startled to see a light-colored circle over twelve inches in diameter in the black fiberglass lining close to the coil. I took a sample of this material and with my microscope discovered that the entire mass of this circle was *Penicillium* mold. The most likely cause for this growth was moisture droplets released from the coil and deposited on the dirty fiberglass lining.

As these stories illustrate, the biggest danger in central air conditioning systems is water leaking onto surfaces with nutrients. This is why the fiberglass manufacturers' trade association recommends that if fiberglass lining in ducts and air handling units becomes wet, it should be replaced. Water should flow only through the condensate drain line; it should never leak or overflow from a central air conditioning unit. In my opinion fiberglass lining should never be exposed close to a cooling coil, because if the material contains dust nutrients, it is a perfect environment for the growth of microorganisms. In addition, lining that is near the coil and the blower should be made of a nonfibrous material (such as closed-cell foam made for the purpose or foil-covered fiberglass) and have a smooth surface that can be cleaned. Ideally, the interior surface near the cooling coil should be metal, with the

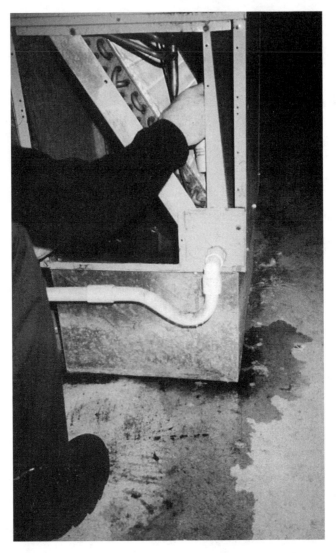

FIGURE 10.6. Leak testing a heat pump condensate tray. The condensate tray at the low side of the heat pump coil was leaking. The water from the tray was supposed to drain out through the white pipe; instead it was dripping into the fiberglass insulation lining the metal box and onto the concrete floor. The woman living in the town house developed respiratory problems and was forced to move out.

insulation sandwiched between the exterior and interior walls of the AHU. In this setup the insulation can never get dirty or wet, and the walls can easily be wiped clean. (All cooling coils should also be fully accessible for cleaning.)

An odor like sweat socks (or any moldy odor, for that matter) coming from the air conditioning system is an indication of biological growth. You may notice this smell is particularly strong when the air conditioning first starts up. This is because air that has been sitting around the contaminated materials near the coil becomes saturated with the smell of mold, bacteria, or yeast and thus contains a higher concentration of the odor. I have sampled the dust in hundreds of air conditioning units and almost always find biological growth, because they contain the two basic elements to support life in air: water and nutrients. Get rid of one or the other and the chances of microbiological growth are greatly reduced.

To prevent accumulation of dust and skin scales on the air conditioning coil and interior surfaces, including the fiberglass lining, use an air filter with a minimum of 40 percent efficiency and change the filter at least twice a season. If you run your AHU most of the year, you may want to change the filter more often. *The typical fiberglass "furnace filters" used in air conditioning systems are completely inadequate, and in my opinion they are responsible for a significant percentage of IAQ problems.*

Reducing Moisture and Nutrients

I cannot state this strongly enough: If you have central air conditioning, it is essential that you keep the interior of the AHU completely dust-free. Vacuuming contaminated insulation, as I have often seen attempted, is not a solution, because the organisms causing the trouble are deep within. In addition, vacuuming with a non-HEPA vacuum can cause additional IAQ problems. If you have a very dirty return duct, have it professionally cleaned as well, because you can't really tell by looking whether the dust is contaminated. (If you are curious, you can send a dust sample to a laboratory for analysis. If you are sensitized, wear an N95 NIOSH mask when handling the dust.) Contaminated lining materials must be replaced, preferably with closed-cell foam or foil-covered fiberglass. If you are sensitized to moldy dust the work should be done by a professional, and great caution should be used during both cleaning and removal of contaminated materials.

The location of a duct can determine the extent of biological growth. If a ceiling return grille is in a hallway just outside a bathroom, for example, warm, moist air will rise by convection through the grille and into the duct when the bathroom door is opened after someone showers. In cold weather this moisture will condense in the dust on the walls inside the duct, and mold will grow. I have seen such returns, and in at least two houses I found that almost half the dust in the return duct consisted of growing fungi—*Alternaria* in one home and *Cladosporium* in the other. Children with significant allergy and asthma symptoms were living in both homes. The solution is not to keep the bathroom door closed after a shower (see chapter 4) but to seal the return grille in the seasons when the air conditioning system is not running. The simplest way to do this is to wrap aluminum foil around a new filter and place it inside the grille. If you are planning to install air conditioning with the air handling unit in the attic, don't place the return near a bathroom! Remember, too, that if a return duct or any duct runs through an unheated attic, the duct will be cooled in winter, which can lead to condensation. (For more information on air handling units and attics, see chapter 12.)

One HVAC contractor in Minnesota described an odor problem in a home with an attic air handling unit and flexible ducts. The supply ducts for the AHU rested on the attic floor joists in a wavelike pattern. At the top of the joists the ducts were supported, but in the space between them the ducts drooped. The contractor told me he had removed gallons of water from these ducts. Apparently warm, moist air from the house rose by convection into the ducts, and water condensed and accumulated at the bottoms of the loops. If you have an AHU in the attic, be sure to close or seal all the ceiling registers in the colder months when the air conditioning is not operating to keep out warm, moist air. Insulated metal ducts are preferable to flexible plastic ones.

I have heard that some people living where it is hot and dry in the summer use "swamp coolers" for cooling the air. I've never seen such a system, but I've been told it consists of a water reservoir with an evaporative pad and a blower. The same principles apply wherever there are nutrients and water in air. The airflow in a swamp cooler has to be completely free of dust if microbiological growth is to be avoided.

Reducing Moisture by Dehumidifying Air

One of the paradoxes of air conditioning is that the system blows cold air that is saturated with moisture. Ideally we would like an air conditioning system to produce cool, dry air. This is difficult to achieve, however, because as the air temperature drops the relative humidity rises. As air passes over a cooling coil, moisture condenses, but the air remains cold and at its dew point.

Is there any way to reduce relative humidity and thus moisture within an air conditioning system? Before the energy crisis of the 1970s, electric heaters were used in commercial systems to warm the air after it passed over the coil and thus to lower the relative humidity. But cooling and then slightly warming the air was such a waste of energy that the practice was abandoned. A more efficient way to do this is to use an air-to-air heat exchanger and take heat from the incoming air to raise the temperature of the air leaving the cooling coil a few degrees. This method is used in some dehumidifying equipment.

Most people with central air conditioning don't have this kind of equipment. Ultimately air conditioning systems should be controlled by both relative humidity (with a "dehumidistat") and temperature (with a thermostat) rather than by temperature alone. As far as I know this approach is not in common use. Until dehumidistats have some control over our spaces, if your air conditioning thermostat is set at 70°F, it will turn off at that temperature even if the relative humidity is 80 percent, which would still be uncomfortably humid and conducive to mold growth.

Central air conditioning provides great relief not only to those who live in hot, humid climates, but also to the many individuals with asthma or allergies to pollen and mold. If someone in your family has such problems and you can choose the kind of system installed in your home, I recommend avoiding hot-air heat with central air conditioning.

DUCTS

- Ducts should not run through concrete.
- Ducts should not be caked with dust.
- Hire professionals to clean your ducts, and be sure they take great care not to spread the irritants into the air. When the ducts are cleaned, have the blower cabinet and blower (as well as the air conditioning coil, if there is one) cleaned of all dust.
- If the fiberglass insulation lining your air handling unit (heat pump, furnace, or air conditioner) or ducts has gotten wet or is moldy, have it replaced. Be careful that contaminants are not spread into the air while the work is being done. I encourage the use of either nonfibrous insulation or fiberglass covered with aluminum foil.
- If you have fiberglass ducts in your home that have become contaminated, replace them.
- If flexible ducts have become contaminated, consider replacing those that are accessible.
- Inspect the ducts by removing a register and looking in with a mirror and flashlight.
- Don't use biocides and adhesive sprays in ducts.
- Avoid return systems with panned bays.
- Be sure your return is properly ducted and airtight.

FILTRATION

- If possible, do not use inexpensive fiberglass filters. Use the most efficient filter available for your system, to prevent dust accumulation. If you can, use throwaway media filters, not washable types.
- I don't recommend electronic filters, because they have to be cleaned at least monthly.
- I also do not recommend electrostatic filters because they too have to be cleaned.

HUMIDIFIERS

- Do not install a furnace humidifier.
- If you have a furnace humidifier, get rid of it if there is a tray full of water.
- If you must have a humidifier, use a steam or trickle type (see chapter 3).

AIR CONDITIONING

- If there is any debris on an air conditioning coil, have the coil professionally cleaned and disinfected.
- Be sure the condensate pan is not leaking, and have it cleaned regularly by a technician. Check that the condensate line has a trap and that it is not clogged.
- Don't place the air return grille in the hall ceiling outside a bathroom.
- If the air handling unit is in the attic, seal all duct openings (return and supply registers) during the colder months when the air conditioning is not operating.
- Window air conditioners can also become contaminated with growth; refer to the recommendations at the end of chapter 3.

MISCELLANEOUS

- Install carbon monoxide detectors in your home. Follow the manufacturer's instructions for installation and maintenance.

CHAPTER

11

More on Heat and Fuel

When people live in cold climates, they have to heat their homes. The kind of horror stories you'll read in this chapter can almost always be avoided by engaging qualified professionals to maintain your heating system conscientiously and by using common sense in monitoring the equipment. Chapter 10 focused on hot-air heating and on cooling systems; this chapter covers electric, hot-water, and steam heat as well as water heaters and fuel.

BASEBOARD HEATERS

Baseboard electric convectors work rather like toasters. Neither has a motor, and both have metal filaments that heat up when electricity passes through them. Both are also very low maintenance, but the high temperatures they generate can cause fires. For example, curtains can be scorched if they touch electric baseboard heaters. In one basement apartment I found an extension cord resting on the heater. All the cord's insulation had melted at one spot, and the cord was stuck to the heater's metal cover. If the metal hadn't been painted, supplying a thin layer of insulation, a short circuit could have started a fire. Electric baseboard heaters can be a particular worry in children's rooms, where plastic toys and other combustibles may end up near or inside the heating unit. On one home inspection I found the child's pillow on top of the heater.

During an air quality inspection in a finished basement, I saw an open door that was completely flush with the front of a baseboard heater. Apparently the

190

door was always kept open. As I started to close it, smoke rose from a blackened band of charcoal at the bottom where the wood was smoldering.

Why hadn't the owners noticed the problem? To answer, I have to describe the burning process. In chapter 5 we looked at the thermal decomposition of wood, which produces combustible vapors. When wood burns with a flame, it is these vapors that are burning and that supply the energy to decompose more wood. But wood can decompose without a flame when enough heat energy is supplied. Three ingredients are required for wood to burn with a flame: an ignition source, sufficient heat, and enough oxygen. "Burning" is the chemical combination of oxygen with carbon-containing materials. The more oxygen there is, the faster the chemical changes take place. With an increased rate of chemical change, more heat is produced and therefore higher temperatures are reached.

Think about a fireplace. You arrange the wood and light the logs, but sometimes the "fire" smolders rather than burns. Smoke is produced (more smoke than when the fire is burning, and remember, smoke is toxic), but there is no flame. If you pick up a bellows and blow air onto a glowing embers, a flame appears because the increased flow of oxygen speeds up the chemical change and thus increases the temperature. If you try to burn wet wood the fire may also smolder, because some of the heat is being spent on evaporating the moisture within the cellulose structure rather than fueling thermal decomposition.

When I started to close the door in this basement, I moved the wood at the bottom of the door away from the baseboard heater, introducing more oxygen to the heated wood surface. The rate of chemical change in the wood increased, producing smoke. If you have baseboard electric heat or supplementary electric heat in any room in your house, be sure nothing combustible ever comes in contact with the heaters.

BOILERS

As a home inspector, I am always amused when people refer to a boiler as a furnace. A furnace heats air; a boiler heats water. Both can use either gas or oil for fuel, depending on the type of burner. Inside a gas-fired boiler or furnace, the burners produce a gas flame, not very different from that on a gas stove. On an oil-fired boiler or furnace, a burner pumps a very fine mist of oil into a stream of air moving from a blower into the combustion chamber. An electric spark from a transformer ignites the mixture of fuel and air.

The mist is an aerosol of microscopic oil droplets that forms as the liquid is sprayed through a small hole or slit in a nozzle. As long as the opening is smooth and clean, the shape of the spray is straight and symmetrical. If the nozzle is dirty or clogged, the mist may point to the side rather than to the middle of the combustion chamber. The flame may then touch the sides of the chamber, resulting in incomplete combustion and producing soot (see chapter 5).

There are two kinds of boilers. The most common type is a forced hot-water boiler, in which water is heated and then circulated through radiators or baseboard convectors or, in the case of radiant heat, through tubing in the floor. The less common type, a steam boiler, boils the water and turns it to water vapor ("steam"), which then travels through pipes into radiators.

Radiators and baseboard convectors can be a source of allergens and irritants, particularly if they have never been cleaned or if previous owners had mold or mite problems or kept pets. In many homes where inhabitants were suffering from allergies, the rooms seemed spotless, yet I found thick clumps of dust either between the radiator coils or on the bottoms of baseboard convectors. (A baseboard convector consists of a cover with a louver at the top and fin tubing inside.) In two homes where the owners had chronic coughs, *Aspergillus* mold was growing in the accumulated dust stuck to the fin tubing inside.

I inspected one home after a young family had purchased it and had the lead paint professionally abated. The mother, who was allergic to mold and mites, and baby were fine when they visited the house before buying it. When they entered the vacant house after having the lead paint removed, the mother experienced respiratory distress and the baby became ill. Two weeks later, after recovering, the mother returned alone to the still vacant house for twenty minutes, to see if she would react. Hours after her brief visit, she became hoarse and could barely speak for several days. The family postponed their move and feared they would have to sell the house.

Even though most of the home had been thoroughly cleaned by the lead removal contractor, I found the radiators had a thick layer of ancient accumulated dust. With a microscope I could see large numbers of mite fecal pellets

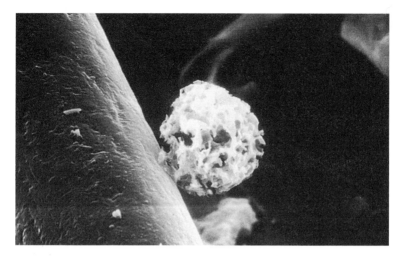

FIGURE 11.1. Oil soot on a synthetic carpet fiber. This soot particle looks like a hollowed-out golf ball. Such spheres, which consist of soot (carbon) and unburned fuel, can often be found in the winter in both exterior and interior air. (4,000× SEM)

and pet dander in the dust. Apparently the previous owner's housekeeping efforts had not been prizewinning. Why didn't the mother's symptoms appear before the lead cleanup? My guess is that to "protect" the radiators from the lead dust generated during the abatement, the workmen covered them with plastic. When the covers were removed, the irritating dust in the radiators was disturbed and became aerosolized. On one radiator I could see a large fingertip-shaped depression in the dust layer! The woman called me several weeks later to say she was able to live in the house once the remaining carpets had been removed and the radiators cleaned with a HEPA vacuum and "dry" steam to destroy allergens.

If anyone in your family has allergies, be sure to clean the heat sources thoroughly, not only before you move into the home but every year before you turn the heat on for the season. This is harder than it seems, because the spaces in many radiators are not very accessible. An inexpensive special vacuum attachment makes the job possible, however (see the resource guide at the end of the book). Radiators sometimes have metal covers, and the removable plates on baseboard convectors can be stuck on by paint. If a radiator or baseboard is covered, remove the cover to clean the pipes or fin tubing.

Boiler Neglect

When houses were heated with fireplaces and coal stoves, people knew they were dealing with fire. With the advent of central heat, however, the flame moved into the basement, out of sight and thus out of mind. Rather than throw a log on the fire or shovel coal into the stove, all they had to do was turn up the thermostat. Because heating equipment is now generally hidden away (and we don't have to remove the ashes), more often than not it is neglected.

One man who was selling his house had called the gas company several times because he smelled something in the finished basement where his children often played. When I entered with the real estate agent and prospective buyer on the prepurchase inspection, I noticed the odor of combustion gases the moment I went down into the basement. I was concerned, because combustion gases may contain carbon monoxide (CO). As I inspected the boiler, I made a point of kneeling to avoid breathing hazardous gases that I suspected were hanging in an invisible cloud below the ceiling.

I looked with a mirror and a flashlight to see if combustion gases were leaking out of the boiler. Combustion gases from a gas flame contain over 50 percent water vapor, and when the hot gases hit a cold mirror, the moisture condenses just as it does when you breathe on a mirror, when your glasses fog up on coming inside on a cold winter day, or when you leave an air conditioned room and walk out into humid, hot air. In all these cases moisture from the air condenses onto cooler surfaces because they are below the dew point.

The mirror fogged when I held it near the combustion chamber, so I decided to measure the concentration of carbon monoxide in the basement with my Bacharach Monoxor II. The concentration was elevated at the ceiling, about twenty parts of carbon monoxide per million parts of air (20 ppm). In a house the CO concentration should not exceed 9 ppm, but normally the concentration is zero. Even at 9 ppm—the "acceptable" level—people who are sensitive to combustion products may feel sick. And it isn't just the carbon monoxide that is unhealthy; combustion gases without CO present can also cause symptoms because they too are toxic.

As soon as I completed my measurement, the real estate agent, who was quite tall and had been standing next to me, left the basement for some fresh outdoor air. You might think the seller would have been upset by my findings, but in fact he was elated, because at last he knew his worry about the odor in the basement was justified.

It didn't cost a lot to fix this serious problem. The gas pressure had to be adjusted at the control, and accumulated rust chips that had fallen from the heat exchanger had to be removed from the gas burners. The excessive gas pressure and the rust chips had distorted the flame, resulting in incomplete combustion. If there is rust on the burners or on the exterior case of your boiler, the boiler may need maintenance. More often than not, rust on the outside is a sign of a water leakage. Water should never be leaking from a boiler that is operating properly. If you see water, don't just put a pot there as I have seen so many homeowners do. Have the leak fixed.

In one home a simple boiler leak led to mildew and occupant allergies. I was asked to investigate the home because the owner was concerned about the lack of heat to the bedroom radiators and the moisture that condensed on the second-floor windows in the winter. I found water dripping from the boiler circulator. As water leaked out, air entered the system and found its way to the bedroom radiators. When the radiators became fully air bound, hot water could not circulate through them, and the bedrooms stayed cold. The low bedroom temperature led to mildew growth on the exterior walls. This condition had been a problem for fifteen years, and the amount of rust around the leak site confirmed this. In addition, the water that dribbled out of the boiler all evaporated into a relatively small crawl space. This moist air infiltrated the home from the space and condensed on the windows. Mites foraged in the mildew in the closets and along the bedroom baseboards.

Know where your boiler shutoff valve is located, so that if it leaks you can turn off the water supply. If you have radiant heating, in which the piping is looped within the flooring, be sure you know where to find the shutoffs for the boiler and loops. Since the loops are not visible and many are plastic, be sure to check periodically under floors for leaks (where possible).

Because the flame is sootier, oil-fired boilers always require more attention and maintenance than those that burn gas. The combustion chamber and heat exchanger inside an oil boiler need inspection and cleaning at least annually. I often find boilers that have not been serviced for several years. When such a boiler fires up, smoke and sometimes even red-hot, glowing bits of soot can blow out of the front of the case. When I shut down the burner in a boiler and look into the observation door with a mirror and a flashlight, I sometimes find that the heat exchanger "passageways" are completely blocked by rust, fuel impurities, and debris deposited from the ceramic combustion chamber liner. When the passageways are blocked like this, there is barely any chimney draft. The combustion products have to go somewhere, and they often end up in the basement.

Most people who burn oil have service contracts with their oil delivery companies for annual maintenance. Unfortunately the annual "cleaning" usually entails only replacing the oil filter and the burner nozzle. The heat exchanger passageways may get cleaned only when a homeowner complains about soot or odors. If you have oil combustion equipment, be sure the interior of the heat exchanger is inspected annually and is brush cleaned at least every other year.

In one apartment building the oil-fired boiler had not been adequately serviced. My client, a young mother, was living on the second floor. The large boiler was confined in a small mechanical room in the basement. Soot and a strange odor were entering the woman's apartment, and ever since quitting her job to stay home with a new baby, she had had a strange taste in her mouth, a dry throat, and frequent headaches—all of which seemed worse in the winter.

The management company had attempted to solve the problem by lining the chimney—an expensive procedure. They were also planning to rebuild both the walls abutting the chimney in the woman's apartment and the walls in the apartment below, where another tenant had similar complaints. When I inspected the boiler, I could see that there was delayed ignition—the oil burner was firing too long before the spark ignited the fuel. This allowed the oil mist to build up in the combustion chamber so that when the flame hit it a small explosion ensued, characterized by a thumping "whoosh!" In the confined space of a combustion chamber, an explosion creates excessive pressure, driving combustion products and unburned fuel droplets outward. When this type of explosion produces black clouds (owing to incomplete combustion of the fuel), it is referred to as a puff-back. A puff-back can blow the observation door off a boiler or fill an entire building with soot. The cleanup from puff-backs can be very costly, but it is usually covered by homeowners' insurance.

After spending about twenty minutes in the smoky mechanical room, I too got a headache and had a metallic taste in my mouth—exactly the same symptoms my client had experienced. The management company had the burner serviced and adjusted so that the fuel ignited sooner, and that relieved the condition in both apartments.

To check for delayed combustion, it's a good idea to watch your boiler when it first ignites. Don't stand too close, however, as I learned on one inspection! When a commercial gas boiler with delayed ignition lit while I was standing nearby, my pants were engulfed in the burner flame. Fortunately the flame rollout was brief and was not hot enough to set fire to my trousers. On another home inspection the buyer and I were trapped in a low crawl space in front of the horizontally mounted furnace. I had pointed out the location of the emergency power shutoff switch and was explaining how to change the furnace filter when the broker raised the thermostat. As the gas-fired furnace ignited, the flame rollout was so huge that the floor joists above were engulfed in the flame. I was so terrified that the buyer had to remind me where to find the shutoff switch.

Whether your burner uses gas or oil, I recommend you purchase a service contract and have your mechanical equipment inspected annually. (And have a carbon monoxide detector installed.) One last observation that may seem ridiculous: Boilers have fires inside, and the metal vent pipe from the boiler to the chimney can be extremely hot, in some cases over 400°F. I often find the instruction booklet lying on top of the boiler case, in direct contact with the vent pipe. Such booklets are often scorched (making them difficult to read). I tell everyone who has a boiler to make sure there is nothing combustible within three feet of the equipment.

Direct-Vented Boilers

In traditional boilers and furnaces, hot combustion gases are vented through metal pipes into the chimney flue, where natural draft draws the gases to the exterior. Some newer combustion equipment is vented directly to the exterior through plastic piping. This type of equipment does not depend on natural draft to draw out the combustion gases; instead, a blower pulls the gases out of the combustion chamber and pushes them through the vent piping to the exterior.

I have found two problems with this kind of equipment. In many homes the vent pipe joints are not airtight, and because the gases are under pressure, they stream into the house air. Even when the pipe joints are airtight the house itself is not, and combustion gases can leak back into the house (infiltrate) through leaky windows and openings in the foundation or around the vent pipe itself. (When combustion gases exit through a chimney, they enter the air above the roof and from there rise into the atmosphere.)

I have had a number of clients who became ill when combustion gases spilled from direct-vented equipment. I feel strongly that oil-fired equipment should not be direct vented through the side of the house, because the combustion products have a powerful odor that usually finds its way back in.

One family I worked with had a direct-vented, gas-fired boiler in the basement, and the chimney was no longer being used. I found that large amounts of combustion gases, which contain moisture, were leaking into the house from the vent piping as well as from outside through the wall gap around the vent pipe itself. I recommended they vent the boiler back into the chimney flue, if allowed by the manufacturer. When I called several weeks later to see if they had noticed an improvement in the air quality, they said the only difference was that the air was so dry their daughter's hair became charged with static electricity when she brushed it. The family may have been missing the moisture, but I knew their indoor environment was a lot healthier without the combustion gases!

STEAM DISTRIBUTION

When the boiler in a steam heating system is not running, the radiators and pipes are full of air. When the boiler has been running for some time and the radiators are hot, all the pipes and radiators are full of water vapor. Thus there must be some mechanism to allow for airflow in and out of the system as the boiler cycles on and off.

Most steam radiators have a shiny metal air vent at the side, allowing air to bleed out of the system as the water vapor is arriving and into the system as the vapor condenses when the radiator cools. The air vents are small but essential components of a steam heating system.

If an air vent isn't working properly, it's either stuck open or stuck shut. If the vent is stuck open, steam pours into the house in a steady stream, condenses on nearby surfaces, and may cause wood floors to decay, paint or wallpaper to peel, and mold to grow near the radiators. In some homes many of the vents leak so badly that the paint on the outside of the house is peeling as well. On the other hand, if the vent is stuck shut, water vapor will not be able to enter that radiator, and the room will lose its heat source.

I have been in homes where, for this very reason, only one or two radiators were working. If the thermostat is in a room with insufficient heat, the boiler runs almost continuously trying to heat the air up to the "set point," the temperature set on the thermostat. This wastes a lot of fuel. Although a thermostat has temperature gradations, the burner on any boiler can only be either on or off. When you turn the thermostat up, the burner ignites. When the air near the thermostat reaches the temperature you have set, the burner turns off. Where all radiators are working, a large volume of vapor is circulating throughout the system and air in every heated room is warmed. In a house where, say, only two of ten radiators are working because the air vents on the others are stuck shut, much less vapor circulates. It takes much longer for the two radiators to warm the air enough to reach the thermostat temperature setting. During this time the burner in the boiler is firing and burning fuel. Much of the heat being generated is going up the chimney instead of making steam for the radiators, and the resulting combustion gases are that much hotter.

Air Vent Phantoms

Even properly operating air vents can be sources of irritants. I was once asked by a housing agency to determine why a new boiler was making an elderly occupant feel ill. She complained of a sickening odor, and even though carbon monoxide is odorless, the fire department had tested for it and found none. The situation had become serious: the woman's family was demanding that the new $4,000 boiler be replaced. Obviously the housing authority, which had subsidized the boiler's installation, hoped to avoid this expense.

When I arrived, quite a crowd was waiting for me: the woman, two of her grown children, their attorney, the plumber who had installed the boiler, and representatives from the housing authority and the boiler manufacturer. It was tough for the whole group to crowd into the basement, but we managed. I sensed a lot of hostility. The woman's children were very upset, because neither the installer nor the manufacturer would believe anything was wrong, and the installer and the manufacturer suspected the woman was imagining the smell.

I found nothing unusual about the boiler or its installation. Next I went to look at the distribution system—the radiators. I went upstairs and, as the water vapor was about to arrive, held a clean glass upside down over the air vent of the dining room radiator while air was exiting. I quickly inverted the glass and took a sniff. There was a fleeting odor of heated rubber. I repeated the test and asked the woman to take a sniff. She immediately recognized the smell that had been making her sick. The manufacturer's representative said there was a rubber gasket in the boiler, and I think it must have been off-gassing when it was heated.

I recommended the housing authority attach small plastic tubes to each of the air vents and lead them outside through holes in the walls. In this arrangement, whenever the water vapor entered the radiators it would push the smelly air outside the home rather than into the rooms. Those little plastic tubes saved the housing authority a lot of money, and I suspect that once the gasket stopped smelling they were able to remove them. In the meantime, I heard from the housing authority representative that the house looked and sounded like a teakettle as vapor puffing from the tubes condensed to steam in the cold exterior air.

Earlier in the chapter I referred to water vapor in heating pipes as steam, or water in its gaseous state. Unfortunately "steam" has two meanings in common usage: water vapor (the gaseous state) in a pipe and water droplets (the liquid state) suspended in air. When liquid water is boiled, it becomes vapor inside the heating pipes; when the vapor is released through the radiator air vent, it condenses into droplets in the cooler room air. In chapter 4 I mentioned that water vapor is not visible but that suspended droplets of water are, because they reflect light. This is why the vapor released into the outside air made the house look like a steaming teakettle.

In this case only the woman herself was bothered by the smell. Other emissions from steam air vents can affect more people. In one apartment building a chemical had been added to the boiler water to minimize corrosion. This chemical, called an amine, can cause skin irritation. A small amount of it evaporated into the air within the heating system, and when the water started to boil and steam moved through the pipes, this air was pushed out the vents. Some people in the building found it irritating.

Pipe Poltergeists

A steam heating system sometimes makes banging and hissing noises that sound as if a ghost is trapped inside. The hissing is caused by the air vents as they cool periodically and let steam out. The banging is produced when hot-water vapor (the gas in the pipe) encounters cooler, condensed water in radiators or pipe elbows. As it cools from the contact, the vapor condenses from a gas to a liquid, which takes up less space. The water implodes as it rushes in to fill the space that had been taken up by the vapor. In the process, the water hits itself and the interior walls of the pipes. The energy from the impact causes vibrations that we perceive as sound, which are transmitted along the pipes or radiator.

A properly constructed steam distribution system is designed so that all the condensate water from the radiators and pipes will flow back to the boiler without leaving behind any pools of water. If radiators are not pitched properly, toward the valve, a puddle accumulates at the bottom of the radiator, creating conditions that lead to the banging noise. Banging can be produced anywhere within the system where water accumulates, but the noise is most likely to occur in two places: at an elbow somewhere in the pipe system where the angle is less than ninety degrees, or at the valve at the bottom of the radiator.

People tell me that banging radiators have kept them awake at night through most of the winter. If you have noisy radiators, you may only need to place two small wooden shims under the radiator legs to alter the slope. Another hint: be sure the valve at the bottom of the radiator is opened all the way, to give lots of room for the vapor to enter and the condensate water to drain back into the pipe.

WATER HEATERS

There are several ways to use a boiler to heat water for domestic use. In a tankless coil, water piping passes through the boiler itself. In an indirectly fired water heater, water from the boiler is pumped through a coil of piping inside a large water storage tank. The principle is similar in both types, but in one the coil is inside the boiler and the water that goes through it is the domestic hot water. In the other type the coil is in a separate tank, and the water going through the coil is boiler water, not domestic hot water. In tankless coils, mineral deposits accumulate on the inside walls of the tubing, restricting the flow of hot water. In the indirectly fired system, minerals can build up in the water tank on the outside of the coils, but this will not restrict the flow.

If your hot water is supplied in any way by your boiler, then the boiler is running all year round and there is some heat loss from it to the basement, even if the boiler is insulated. In basements of homes with tankless coils or indirect fired heaters, I usually find significantly less mildew because the basements are warmer and the relative humidity is thus lower during the summer.

The most common kind of water heater is a separate tank fired by oil, gas, or electricity, which is the most expensive energy source. The biggest drawback I find with fuel-burning water heaters is spillage of combustion gases caused by inadequate chimney draft. In fact, in some newer homes with high-efficiency heating systems, blowers are installed to eliminate the combustion products. If the heating system and the water heater share a common vent pipe and the chimney draft is inadequate, combustion gases from the furnace or boiler can be blown out the water heater vent pipe into the basement air. The situation is more likely in a gas-fired water heater than in an oil-fired one, because there is an opening at the top of a gas water heater. The opening, called a *draft diverter,* is there to prevent downdrafts from blowing out the pilot light. Combustion gases from a boiler or furnace can exit through this opening. (This problem does not occur with an electric water heater because it doesn't burn anything and therefore doesn't need to be vented.)

The combustion chamber in a gas-fired water heater is at the bottom, where there is an access cover. I have seen many gas-fired water heaters that malfunctioned because of blockages in the vent system, allowing hot combustion gases to exit at the access. The temperature was so high that it melted the plastic knobs on nearby valves. The same caution thus applies to vented water heaters as to boilers and furnaces: don't place combustibles nearby.

Legionnaires' Disease

If your water heater is a great distance from your bathroom, you may get impatient or annoyed waiting for hot water to arrive. But imagine how long you would have to wait in a large hotel, hospital, or apartment building, where the water heater is many floors away, if such buildings used the same kind of system used in a home. In a typical single-pipe residential system, you have to wait because the water that has cooled is sitting in the pipe and has to be pushed out before the fresh hot water arrives. To avoid this delay, a few big homes and most larger buildings have a "two-pipe" system for the hot water. In this type of a system a pump continuously circulates the hot water through a long "loop" of piping that runs throughout the building. Each fixture is attached to the loop. As soon as you open your hot faucet, water from the loop exits the spout.

The two-pipe system solves one problem but may create another. The bacteria called *Legionella* that cause Legionnaires' disease grow best in constantly warm water, optimally about 105°F. In residential hot-water pipes, the temperature fluctuates from hot to room temperature with usage, but in larger buildings, with two-pipe hot-water systems, the temperature in the piping remains relatively constant, allowing *Legionella* to proliferate in the biofilms that adhere to interior surfaces of pipes and fixtures. People with compromised immune systems are more susceptible to all diseases, and some of them may have contracted Legionnaires' disease while showering when they were patients in a hospital. Legionnaires' disease has also infected people staying in large hotels. (Owners of buildings with two-pipe systems should probably periodically have the hot water tested for *Legionella*.)

Leakage

One problem common to all types of water heaters is leakage, both slow and catastrophic. Slow leaks can cause all kinds of mold growth, depending on where the leak is and how long it has been occurring. I recommend that homeowners check their tanks for leaks at least weekly. When a water heater breaks, cold water flows uncontrolled into the basement, mechanical closet, or wherever the water heater is. This can destroy a house. Make sure you know where the shutoff valve for your water heater is, and use it if the heater breaks (but turn the fuel or power supply off first). When water heaters are in living spaces such as finished basements or in mechanical closets in apartments, I recommend adding an overflow pan with a floor water alarm. Some hardware stores carry these alarms; you can also find distributors of these devices on the Internet.

Water heaters come with either a five- or a ten-year warranty. The difference between the two warranties has nothing to do with the quality or construction of the tank. A water tank contains either one or two magnesium rods, which protect the tank from corrosion in the same way that a zinc coating protects a galvanized nail from rusting. Over time the magnesium rod dissolves. If a heater has one rod, the lifetime under typical water conditions is five years; with two rods, it's ten years. Be sure to check your warranty and consider replacing your water heater if it's well beyond its warranty life, or you may come home one day and find your basement full of water.

If you are going to be away from home for a time, ask a friend or neighbor to keep an eye on your boiler and water heater. Make sure this person is reliable. One of my clients made the mistake of asking the wrong person to watch her house while she was away for the winter. Something went wrong with the boiler and the heat went off. Pipes burst and flooded the house. When the woman returned the entire house was wet, and a soggy bill for thirty thousand gallons of water was waiting for her. Mold was growing on the living room couch, the bedroom lamps, and all the interior walls. Ceilings had collapsed, and the recently refinished wood floors were so buckled and warped from swelling that they looked like frozen waves. The house was "totaled" and is scheduled to be gutted and completely renovated.

Fortunately the damage was covered by her insurance policy.

FUEL PROBLEMS

Oil spills are pungent and dangerous to health. One young woman made an offer on a split-level home with a finished basement. On her first visit to the house she noticed a solvent smell, but she ignored it because the property seemed so perfect for her. The house had just been painted, so she assumed the paint might be causing the smell.

Six months after she moved in the solvent smell still lingered and the woman began having respiratory trouble. In the middle of her first winter in the house, the heating system ran out of oil. The oil company came and filled the tank, but a few days later the tank was empty again. She then made the connection between the solvent smell and the bottomless oil tank.

Apparently there was a pinhole leak in the oil line that had been installed beneath the concrete slab in the basement. Oil had been leaking out for years under the basement floor, and the rate of the leak had clearly increased. Oil had even spread into the well water. Many steps were taken to try to eradicate this nightmare. The basement was excavated about eight feet down, and hundreds of gallons of oil and barrels of saturated soil were removed. The contamination was so widespread, however, that a complete cleanup was impossible. To minimize the chance that the oil remaining in the soil under the house would cause fumes in the occupied space, a radon mitigation system was installed in the basement.

Many of the numerous mitigation steps were necessary, but many mistakes were also made. First, not enough of the contaminated soil was removed. Second, open drums of oil and soil were left in the basement, where they off-gassed fumes into the air. Third, the fan in the radon mitigation system had a leak and the fittings for the pipe to the outside were loose. Instead of blowing the air through the pipe to the roof and the exterior, the system was sucking air laden with oil fumes out of the soil, and some entered the house, making the situation even worse.

What happened to the house was sad, but what happened to the owner was a tragedy. She had originally bought the house in part because it had a basement office. She wanted to work where she lived, not only for convenience but to avoid paying rent for a separate office space. To minimize her mortgage payments, she had put all her savings into the down payment when she bought the house. She originally called me because her home made her feel sick, but she grew so ill from inhaling the oil fumes that she became chemically sensitive and had difficulty working. The insurance company initially refused to pay for a proper oil cleanup, and because she was afraid of losing the house she continued to pay her mortgage even though her income was drastically reduced and she could no longer spend time there.

She decided to sue the insurance company, and her attorney asked me to return and investigate the conditions; by this time two years had passed. To track the levels of contamination in the soil beneath the slab, the mitigation company had installed a "monitoring well" in the basement—a vertical plastic pipe placed in a hole dug down to the water table. I unscrewed the cap to this well and dropped in a small glass vial attached to a six-foot string. When I raised the vial I saw a layer of oil floating on top of the water. In the end the owner and the insurance company reached a settlement so that she was able to buy another house. I hope her new house has gas heat.

Striking Oil

Another homeowner looked out her kitchen window and, to her dismay, saw an oil geyser so high she couldn't see the top. She rushed outside to where the oil truck was parked as it delivered the oil and screamed at the driver. The hose from the truck had sprung a leak right in the middle of her yard. Oil was raining down onto her property; it saturated the soil and lay in a film on top of her kiddie pool. This was a serious cleanup problem, but at least the oil was not inside the building (yet) as it is in so many other cases.

The mitigation company came to clean up the sandy soil and, unfortunately, never warned the owner about some precautions she should take during the removal of the contamination. On cleanup day the smell of oil in her house was so strong she opened all the windows and inserted fans to blow "fresh" air into the house. Instead, she sucked in the contaminated dust, which covered the entire interior of her house. Everything—furniture, floors, rugs—was covered with sand and dust coated with oil. I took samples of sand from the basement floor, and even these reeked of fuel oil. The last time I spoke with the family they were living in a trailer on the edge of their property. I never found out what ultimately happened to the house and its occupants.

In another home built into a hill, the basement was at grade level and sliding doors opened to the front and side yards. The oil fill pipe was in the rear to the left of the house. The homeowner noticed that the fuel in his tank was low and called for a delivery. The tank was filled, but unfortunately someone in the oil company's office sent another tanker. The second deliveryman climbed the hill, put the hose nozzle in the fill pipe, and returned to his truck to eat his lunch. The man must have looked up from his sandwich, noticed oil pouring down the hill, and rushed out to turn off the pump. A neighbor saw him frantically trying to climb back up the oily slope to retrieve the hose, but he kept slipping down at each attempt.

No one told the owner about the afternoon's event, and when he entered his basement that evening he noticed a very strong odor of fuel oil. He looked on the floor and there were puddles of oil everywhere. Apparently his lawn was not the only oil-soaked victim: the excessive pressure had caused the oil tank in the basement to burst.

The company cleaned up the oil spill, but the family called me two years afterward because they had all become chemically sensitive. The owner had a home business in the basement, but he could no longer work there because he was bothered so much by the lingering smell of oil. I noticed a very strong odor of oil in the basement when I entered, as well as a one-inch gap between the foundation wall and the floor. Somehow no one realized that oil from the spill had run beneath the slab, and now fumes were entering the basement from the soil through that gap.

If your basement smells of oil, determine the cause and eliminate the source. If oil has leaked into the concrete and the smell remains after the concrete has been washed, don't hesitate to replace the contaminated portion of the slab. If you use oil for fuel, here are a few more suggestions to improve safety and reduce the likelihood of problems. First, check the bottom of your oil tank. If it's difficult to see, use a bright flashlight and a mirror. If you see hanging oil drops and rust stalactites, or signs of repair, insist that the oil company evaluate the condition of the tank. A new tank costs a lot less than cleaning up a basement full of oil. Second, if your oil line is buried in concrete, install a new line in a leak-tight liner. In addition, install an oil safety valve. This allows oil to flow out of the tank only when the burner is calling for fuel. Third, if you have an older tank that is not in use, have it pumped out and removed. It's not a good idea to save an old oil tank thinking you may switch back to oil in the future. Old tanks may have concealed interior rust that is not visible, particularly if they have been sitting for several years with condensed moisture inside. When a tank is removed, be sure the oil fill and vent pipes are taken out at the same time, or your neighbor's oil may accidentally be delivered into your basement.

Buried Oil Tanks

A student from one of my home-buying courses called to tell me about her experience with a buried oil tank. She was moving to Oregon and had used the non-ASHI home inspector the broker recommended. She expressed concern about the asbestos boiler insulation. The inspector stuck a screwdriver into the insulation and flicked off a piece, exclaiming, "You people from out east are too worried about environmental issues." Then she asked him about the buried oil tank in the backyard. "Nothing to worry about," he replied.

She purchased the home while she was still living in Massachusetts and hired a local company to remove the oil tank. On the day of the excavation, she received a long-distance call at work from the excavator saying that the removal would probably cost $2,000 instead of $500. Later the same day she got a second call with a revised estimate of $5,000. Had a more vigilant home inspector done the inspection, he or she might have recommended the buyer have the seller remove the tank before closing.

Removing buried oil tanks can be very expensive if oil has leaked out of the tank into the surrounding soil. I know of removal/remediation jobs that cost over $60,000. Fortunately the odds of having a leaking tank are about one in two hundred. Nonetheless, it's not worth the risk of continuing to use an old buried oil tank or even to have one on your property. In fact in some states, including Massachusetts, the law requires removal of an abandoned buried oil tank. As long as there is no contaminated soil, removal costs should not be exorbitant.

Gas Exposures and Explosions

In this chapter and others I have cited examples of problems related to exposure to low levels of gas and gas combustion products, particularly for people who are chemically sensitive. If you use gas as a fuel, be insistent about having small leaks repaired. If you smell gas, don't think you are imagining it, even if the gas company representative disagrees. If necessary, purchase your own TIF 8800 combustible gas detector and test for gas leaks yourself. (But don't try to make any repairs!)

All combustion products can be unhealthy, and all fuels are potentially dangerous. Gas explosions are probably less common than oil leaks, but the effects can be far more devastating. One chemically sensitive woman asked me to look at her new house because she thought it was making her ill. She told me she had become chemically sensitive after her many surgeries and hospital stays. She had originally been injured because she was blown out of her home in a gas explosion that demolished the house, leaving her disabled and in a coma for over a year. What had caused this disaster? She had lit a cigarette—her last, in fact—after a gas repairman left the cap on a basement gas pipe open.

RECOMMENDATIONS

HEATING AND FUEL SAFETY

- Be sure nothing combustible (including clothing, boxes, and plastic) and no electrical cords come in contact with electric baseboard heaters or boiler vent pipes. Nothing combustible should be placed within three feet of a boiler.
- Do not allow oil tanks or lines to leak. If you have an oil leak, have a professional cleanup. Be sure the odor is gone after the cleanup has been completed.
- If you have an abandoned underground oil tank on your property, have it removed by a professional. If you are still using your old underground oil tank, have it leak tested or removed.
- If your basement oil tank has been removed, be sure the fill pipe and vent pipe have also been eliminated.
- Have someone monitor your home when you are away.

EQUIPMENT AND INSTALLATION

- Don't install direct-vented oil-fired equipment if the vent goes through a side wall.
- Steam radiators should be pitched toward the valve, which should be completely open when the radiator is in use.
- Install a carbon monoxide detector according to the manufacturer's instructions.
- Have an oil safety valve installed, and make sure the oil line is in a leak-tight liner above, not under, the concrete floor.
- In finished spaces, have a floor water alarm installed in an overflow pan for the water heater.
- A water tank with a ten-year warranty is preferable to one with a five-year warranty. It may cost you more, but you will have fewer floods.

MAINTENANCE

- Keep radiators and baseboard convectors free of dust.
- Whether you use oil or gas fuel, have your heating service company check your equipment for carbon monoxide in the basement and in the combustion products. Technicians should also check the exterior condition of the boiler and the interior condition of the combustion chamber.
- Be sure gas burners are free of all rust, and keep heat exchanger passageways clear.
- From a safe distance, watch your heating system as it ignites to be sure there is no flame rollout or smoke.
- Don't paint steam radiator air vents.
- Be sure air vents are functioning properly.
- Make sure you know where to find the water and fuel or power shutoffs for your boiler and water heater.

12

Attics

Your attic is part of your house. Although most of the airflow is upward from the habitable spaces into the attic, there are ways for allergens to reenter the house, and I encourage you to keep the attic as clean and dust-free as possible. I also discourage people from using the attic as living or play space, particularly if they have asthma or allergies.

Inspecting the attic is part of the ASHI Standards of Practice. When you buy a new home, it's important that your home inspector go up into the attic (if it's accessible) to inspect the insulation, ventilation, and roof sheathing and check any attic mechanical equipment. Attics can sometimes hold deadly secrets. I recently heard about a case in which the inspector (not a member of ASHI) did not tell the prospective buyer there was soot on the attic rafters and sheathing, suggesting an earlier fire or puff-back in the house. The extensive damage had been concealed by repairs in the finished areas of the house. The family moved in and suffered from odors and residues of the chemicals that had been used for cleaning. The house was so toxic that ultimately it was destroyed.

As a residential air quality professional, I look for conditions that lead to increased IAQ problems. But I am also a home inspector, and I often find hazardous structural conditions. This chapter describes some of the unsafe conditions I've found in attics. They are just too important to omit.

For example, pull-down attic stairs can be dangerous and, if installed improperly, can even fall out of the ceiling. Sometimes the levers holding the springs are bent so the spring can fall off and injure anyone going up the stairs.

If you have a pull-down attic stairway, I recommend adding guardrails in the attic around the opening so a misstep won't end in a tumble. And any attic stairs should have a handrail.

ATTIC CRITTERS

A couple purchased an older home with wall-to-wall carpeting. The woman had asthma and was allergic to cats—far more so than she had ever realized. After she and her husband moved into the house, her asthma symptoms became so severe that she was hospitalized. Her husband had the carpeting removed in case it contained allergens. The woman was given an epinephrine injection pen before she was discharged. Within twenty-four hours after returning home she began struggling to breathe and went into anaphylactic shock. Her husband saved her life by carrying her outside and administering the epinephrine.

They asked me how they could make the house safe for her. When I visited, air conditioning was being installed, including an air handling unit in the attic, where I found no flooring and old, loose fibrous insulation between the joists. The air conditioning technicians were carelessly storing the ducts and other components on the joists, and the equipment, including the new ducts, was dusted with loose insulation. There were even clumps of insulation inside the yet-to-be connected ducts.

I suspected the old insulation might contain cat dander. In addition to recommending that the insulation be removed (under containment conditions), I told the couple to have the ceiling attic structure HEPA vacuumed and spray painted. The new, unused air conditioning equipment and ducts also had to be cleaned. They had the attic reinsulated with fiberglass batts. After these steps were taken that typical dusty "old house smell" disappeared entirely from the second floor. Old insulation, filled as it often is with years of dust, dead mice, and insects, may cause the unpleasant odor characteristic of the upper levels and attics of so many older homes. The couple also eliminated all the old house dust from the basement and living spaces, and the wife lived in the house symptom-free.

Fiberglass insulation in attics is often littered with mouse droppings. Although the attic may seem very hot and inhospitable to us, it's relatively cooler near the ceiling, where mice burrow below the surface of the insulation and make nests. In some attics there are hundreds of finger-shaped indentations in the insulation. Mouse urine is smelly enough, but add a carcass or two and an attic infested with mice can become really malodorous. Some mouse infestations can be associated with mites or fecal material containing microbiological hazards, such as hantavirus.

My in-laws lived in an old farmhouse in a rural area of New England. When my wife was growing up there were more mice than people in the house. In addition, although the house was very clean, dozens of flies were always buzzing around inside. In the winter my father-in-law would turn the heat down in some of the unused bedrooms, and the flies would lie dormant concealed in the window tracks. When the rooms heated up, the insects would come alive and buzz against the glass. The fly infestation was so widespread that we sometimes found flies wedged inside the layers of folded sheets and towels in the linen closet.

I think their attic must have been the insects' breeding ground, because it was always alive with hundreds of flies. The attic was also home to generations of mice, and the flies were probably laying their eggs in mouse carcasses, which then fed the maggots. I encouraged the family to reduce the fly population by getting rid of the old insulation where the mice lived and making the house airtight to the exterior, but they thought the flies were just part of country living.

Because most attics are isolated and are generally open to the environment in one way or another, many insects (bees, ants, silverfish, and cockroaches) nest either in the insulation or on the framing. One homeowner asked me to help figure out why there was moisture in the attic. I opened the pull-down stairway and ascended. There were insulation batts between the floor joists, and there was no flooring. The batts were installed upside down, with the vapor barrier facing the attic. I poked my finger through the aluminum foil barrier and was able to squeeze water out of the tuft of fiberglass insulation I removed from the hole.

Moisture was rising from several sources in the rooms below: an unvented dryer, several room humidifiers, and the normal everyday activities such as showering, cooking, and even breathing. I noticed many holes in the vapor barrier. The attic did not have adequate ventilation to the exterior, and I suspect that in the winter moisture was condensing on the roof sheathing, dripping from the nails, pooling on top of the vapor barrier, and leaking through rips into the insulation.

I was surprised at how much moisture I found, even though I understood why it was there. But what lay ahead was like a scene from a horror show. As I walked carefully through the tropical attic to the opposite gable end, my attention was drawn to an oval damp spot on the brick chimney where moisture was condensing on the masonry (which must have been below the dew point of the humid attic air). Near the chimney, on top of the vapor barrier, I saw a textured black circle several feet in diameter. As I neared the area I realized it consisted of thousands of carpenter ants, basking motionless in the warm, moist attic atmosphere. I was so unsettled that I quickly tiptoed away, afraid the vibrations from my steps would arouse the hordes and send them scurrying in my direction.

I recommended the owner remove the wet insulation, let the attic dry out, and then have new insulation installed with the vapor-barrier side down. I also suggested sealing any ceiling openings and chases and improving the attic ventilation by installing ridge and soffit vents. The ant nests would be eliminated along with the insulation, and without the damp, hot attic conditions, I doubted new colonies would move in.

Carpenter ants can also be found nesting in soffits (an overhang of the attic) where trim wood is damp from an overflowing gutter or from frequent roof water flows (see chapter 15). Insect pests prefer constant warmth and humidity. One entomologist I know studied cockroach nesting and feeding behavior and found that roaches live in soffits. He also discovered that when the soffits are ventilated, temperature and humidity fluctuate too much for them, so they nest elsewhere. In one experiment, soffits at both sides of a house were infested with roaches. The entomologist installed soffit vents at one side, and before long the roaches abandoned the ventilated side and moved to the more humid, unventilated side. The presence of carpenter ants signals excessive moisture, but a cockroach infestation can cause asthma. Installing soffit vents makes the attic less hospitable to insects and is thus a step toward a healthier house.

Where there is life, there are predators. In the attic of a house in the woods, I found thousands of larval cases stuck to the rafters and sheathing. Apparently some type of moth larva had pupated in the attic and, given the vast food supply, numerous spiders had set up shop. Spiderwebs hung all around, and beneath each web the wood floor planks were spattered with spider droppings. Wearing a Tyvek protective suit and a respirator, I managed to scrape up about an eighth of a teaspoon of spider droppings. I sent them off to an allergist, who was going to test them against the blood serum of a few of his patients to see if their blood reacted to the proteins in the spider fecal material, suggesting allergy. Unfortunately my precious sample was lost, but I remain convinced that these droppings cause allergy symptoms.

Some of the animals that move into attics are larger. I heard about one family who purchased a home that had been abandoned for many years. They spent a great deal of money renovating the interior, but they never investigated their inaccessible attic. After all the work was done, they came home one day and found that the second-floor ceiling in the master bedroom had collapsed under the weight of raccoon droppings.

In an older building with a flat roof, I was inspecting a top-floor apartment for a buyer and didn't think there would be access to the "attic" crawl space. Above the kitchen table, though, was a square hatch. I stood on a ladder, opened the hatch, looked in, and faced a squirrel nest that consisted of several sections of a newspaper shredded and piled up between the ceiling joists. Running through the paper was an electric cable for the kitchen light fixture that had been chewed entirely bare of insulation for about two feet. Littered around the access hole were metal pots and pans that a previous tenant had thrown into the attic for storage. Had one of those pans landed on the bare wires when current was flowing, it would have created a short circuit, igniting the newspaper and possibly burning the house down. The only good thing that can be said of squirrels living in attics is that, unlike raccoons, they leave all their droppings outside.

Bats also live in attics. One home inspector I spoke with ended up paying for a new ceiling. When inspecting the attic, he was "buzzed" by a bat. He ducked, lost his footing, slipped off the ceiling joists (the attic had no flooring), and fell through the plaster ceiling. Luckily he caught himself on a joist before he fell into the room below.

Birds too live in attics. On a prepurchase inspection of a hundred-year-old home, I had completed the entire house except for the attic, and the buyer seemed pleased up to that point. I opened the eaves access door and stepped in. The buyer followed me, and I cautioned him to be very careful where he stepped, since there was no flooring. One misstep and one of us could fall through the ceiling to the bedroom below. As we walked along the joists, our shoes made loud crunching noises; I looked down at what appeared to be white insulation and suddenly realized I was looking at feathers instead of fiberglass. My buyer, who was Spanish, exclaimed, "Caca de pajaro [bird droppings]!" He turned around and, stepping as fast as he could on the joists, got out the access door and raced out of the house. The family who had lived there for decades had apparently not taken good care of the property. The attic window had fallen out, and generations of pigeons had flown in to roost.

Pigeon droppings (guano) may contain *Histoplasma capsulatum*, a parasitic fungus that can cause mild to serious respiratory infections. The droppings contain spores that become airborne when the guano is disturbed. Great caution should be exercised when such spaces are cleaned, because inhaling large amounts of this dust can cause the illness called histoplasmosis. If you have pigeon guano in your attic and are concerned, have a microbiology lab test for *Histoplasma capsulatum*.

A ROOF OVER OUR HEADS

One of my clients had a long-term roof leak, and the water ran down two stories through a wall cavity and soaked her living room wall. She discovered the leak when she removed a picture and found the wallpaper black with mold. I subsequently found the mold to be *Stachybotrys*, which grows in wet cellulose.

We've seen over and over what moisture can do to our living spaces, and naturally the main function of a roof is to keep rainwater out. Most single-family and two-family homes have gable roofs, and the top layer that faces the weather is most often covered with asphalt shingles. These are fastened to wood roof sheathing that is nailed to the attic rafters. The sheathing consists of either wooden planks (typical in older homes), oriented strand board, or plywood.

As roofing shingles age, they weather and crack, and they can leak (see chapter 15). Water can also leak around chimney and pipe penetrations. This moisture can fuel mold decay of the sheathing and rafters. Very often, water will run down the rafters and into a wall, further spreading decay. To minimize the chance of such problems, every homeowner should check the attic for leaks during a heavy rain.

If you put on new roofing, keep in mind that the hammering releases a great deal of dust from the sheathing and rafters. If the sheathing is covered with mildew (and it often is), the dust will contain extensive amounts of mold. In normal circumstances the mildew on attic sheathing does not become airborne and is generally not an IAQ problem in the rooms below, because air from the house flows into the attic and out the roof rather than vice versa. If there is an air conditioning unit or furnace in the attic, be sure it is protected from the dust. Don't leave stored possessions in the attic exposed to the dust while the new shingles are being installed. And last, if you or anyone in your family has allergies or asthma, stay out of the house during the disturbance, since some dust is sure to circulate by convection into the living areas.

Ventilation

The purpose of attic ventilation in the winter is to keep humidity levels low by allowing moist air to leave the attic. In the summer, ventilation lets hot air out. In older homes the sheathing consists of narrow wooden planks that were installed horizontally with gaps between them. These gaps allow air to escape from the attic at the gable ends of the planks. Even if a homeowner does nothing to provide airflows in an older home, enough air leaks in and out of construction gaps to keep moisture levels down. In newer homes, on the other hand, the roof sheathing consists of four-by-eight sheets of plywood that act as barriers to air and vapor flow. The buildup of moisture can cause condensation on the sheathing, leading to extensive growth of mold and delamination of the plywood. If you walk on the roof of a very poorly ventilated attic where the sheathing is decayed, you might fall through.

To provide ventilation, newer homes usually have soffit vents and a ridge vent at the top of the roof. In theory, air enters at the soffit vents, rises owing to convection, and exits through the ridge vent. Unfortunately, theory isn't always proved true in practice. First, wind direction can thwart the intended airflows. Using smoke tube testing, I have observed air exiting instead of entering soffit vents. In addition, some attics, even though they have ridge and soffit vents, are extremely hot in the summer. I believe many of the newer ridge vents just don't permit enough airflow to let the hot air out of the attic.

When ridge vents first became available, they were manufactured with baffles, a strip of metal bent upward at each side of the vent. These helped reduce the air pressure when the wind blew over the vent and thus increased the flow of air out of the attic (the way blowing across the top of a straw in a glass of water reduces the pressure, causing the water to rise in the straw). Some people thought vents with baffles were unsightly, so the baffles were eliminated. In my view this drastically reduced the efficiency of ridge vents. In addition, to be effective at all, ridge vents must be installed over a sheathing gap so that air can move from the attic to the outside. In older homes that have new roofing, I have often found that roofers neglected to cut away the sheathing at the roof peak, beneath the ridge vent. Though the roofers had encouraged the owners to add this new feature, they might as well have left it off, for there was no gap underneath. If you pay a roofer to install a ridge vent, be sure someone cuts away enough of the sheathing beneath the vent to allow for airflow.

A similar shortcut is sometimes attempted when soffit vents are installed, as the following story illustrates. A family purchased a large home in an expensive community near Boston. They had a very thorough home inspection by a member of the American Society of Home Inspectors who was referred by their attorney. The ASHI inspector identified many defects for the buyers, some of which the sellers refused to recognize. The broker recommended another inspector, whose role was to mollify the buyer and the seller with a second opinion. Without even entering the attic, this inspector pronounced the ventilation adequate. I was then asked to provide yet another "second opinion."

The soffit ventilation consisted of continuous strips of louvered aluminum about two inches wide. These would have been adequate except for one thing I observed when I climbed a ladder and looked closely at the soffits. No one had bothered to cut out a strip of wood behind the metal louvers. There were only a few one-inch circular holes, barely enough to provide any soffit ventilation at all.

Continuous soffit vents can provide adequate ventilation, but the wood behind them must be cut away to allow for airflow. I do not recommend installing small circular soffit vents, since they have minimal open space. In addition, more often than not, the first time the exterior trim on a home is painted, the circular vents are painted over and become completely useless. Also, for any type of soffit vent to operate properly, the spaces above these vents should not be blocked by attic insulation. Again, if attics are not adequately ventilated, moisture can accumulate, leading to mold and decay of the sheathing.

One family called me because of chronic moisture in the attic. The sheathing on the north-facing side of the gable roof was covered with black mildew, and in the middle of the winter icicles were hanging and water was dripping from the exposed nail ends. Why was this happening? I found a large opening in the return duct in the basement, which meant much of the supply air for the hot-air furnace came from the basement rather than from the first-floor return. This reduced the pressure in the basement and drew in cold exterior air through a leaky door to the outside. As a consequence, the upstairs of the home was excessively pressurized, since more air was being supplied to the spaces than was being removed by the return. A humidifier on the furnace evaporated almost a gallon of water into the supply air for every hour the furnace operated. Moist, warm air that was being forced into the cold attic from the pressurized house through openings at the pull-down stairs, ceiling fixtures, and probably other obscure framing gaps was condensing on the cooler surfaces. This was the cause of the attic rain.

Ice Damming

A house can lose heat to an attic in other ways too. For example, gaps can exist around an interior chimney or around a plumbing pipe. Light fixtures recessed in the ceiling below the attic floor can leak warm air. House air can also rise through openings around light fixtures and attic pull-down stairs. To minimize opportunities for warm air to leak into an attic, seal openings around the chimney and pipes with fiberglass, construct a foam box large enough to cover the attic pull-down stairs, and be sure there are no other avenues for airflows, such as air conditioning equipment.

An accumulation of warm air in the attic can lead to ice damming by melting the bottom layer of the snow piled on a gable roof. The meltwater runs (invisibly) down the roofing beneath the snowpack until it reaches the soffit, which overhangs the exterior of the house and is therefore cold. There the water freezes and creates a dam of ice, allowing water to build up behind it.

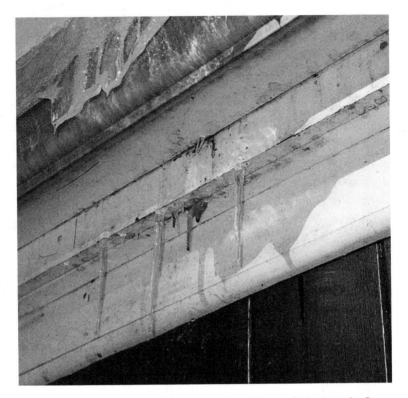

FIGURE 12.1. Ice dam. Ice built up at the edge of this roof, blocking the flow of melting water. The water puddled on the surface of the low-slope roof and leaked under the roofing. The water ran behind the trim and siding, causing staining, peeling, and both visible and concealed wall decay. The homeowners found the mold odor indoors overwhelming.

Roof shingles are not meant to be waterproof but are designed to shed water from the surface. Water building up behind an ice dam gets under the shingles and from there leaks onto the roof sheathing and rafters. In winter, a thick layer of ice in a soffit can sometimes be seen from the attic.

If you do not live in a cold climate, you may never have seen ice damming. You know a house has a problem, however, when you look up and see long icicles hanging from the edge of the roof or gutters. In extreme cases, water from the soffit flows down behind the siding and icicles stick out of the exterior walls. All this ice eventually melts and can cause paint to peel. One ice dam, for example, can cause all the paint to peel off that side of the house. If water enters insulated wall cavities and remains there long enough, the wood can decay. When an ice dam causes indoor leaks, be sure to dry out carpets, walls, or furniture to avoid more serious exposure to mold spores.

I inspected a house in a six-year-old development of eleven homes. As I drove down the street, I noticed that each roof held a thick layer of snow. As I approached the house I was to inspect, I could see that on this particular roof the snow layer was uneven and shallower, and enormous icicles were hanging from the roof edge. I asked the owner what made his house different from the other ten. He said his was the only one with central air conditioning, and the air handling unit was in the attic. The AHU was not airtight, particularly at the filter holder, which had no cover. In the winter, when the air conditioning system was not running, warm air from the house was rising by convection through all the open ceiling diffusers into the air conditioning ducts in the ceiling of the second floor and flowing from the AHU into the attic space. The warmth of the interior air was melting the snow on the roof. As I noted in chapter 10, air conditioning registers should be closed and return ducts sealed during the colder months. That was the solution in this case.

WHOLE-HOUSE FANS

Hot air can also rise from the house into the attic through the louvers of a whole-house fan. This type of fan is normally installed in the second-floor ceiling of a two-story home, with louvers that open with the air flow only when the fan is turned on. A whole-house fan removes 5,000 to 10,000 cubic feet of air per minute from the habitable part of a house and blows it into the attic. From there the air moves outside through the attic vents (gable-end louvers, soffit vents, or ridge vents). When a whole-house fan is working properly, all the air in a typical-sized house is replaced every three to six minutes. But a whole-house fan can be effective only if there are avenues for fresh replacement air to enter and if attic ventilation is sufficient so that the air will flow out of the attic as intended.

I was explaining the operation of a whole-house fan to my buyer on one prepurchase home inspection, warning her that windows had to be open. The seller overheard my remarks and told us about an experience he had one winter evening when he came home from work. As he approached he noticed black smoke pouring out of his attic gable-end louver vents. A fire truck was ahead of him, on its way to the house. All the rooms were full of black smoke. One of his children had accidentally turned on the whole-house fan with all the windows closed. This reduced the air pressure in the house, causing back-drafting at the oil-fired boiler, and the family faced a very costly soot cleanup. Backdrafting can also pull carbon monoxide into a home from a chimney flue. If you have a whole-house fan, I recommend installing a kill switch in the attic so it can't be turned on during the winter. In the summer, always be sure enough windows are open when you operate the fan.

In another home the husband was experiencing allergies related to mold. The finished basement had repeatedly been wet, and the carpeting was con-taminated. The owners were planning to eliminate the carpeting and were keeping the basement door closed until they could do so. In the meantime, however, they used their whole-house fan all summer. I was in the house dur-ing the fall, and the fan was not on, so I asked the woman to set up the house as she normally did in the summer, then turn on the fan. At the second floor they kept one window in every bedroom open, but they did not keep any win-dows open on the first floor. As soon as the fan turned on, the entire first floor smelled of mold. I did a smoke test at the one-inch gap beneath the basement door, and it was obvious that air was billowing from the moldy basement to the first floor when the fan was running.

These two examples illustrate why there has to be a sufficient supply of fresh air in the habitable part of the house when a whole-house fan is oper-ating. This next example shows why there must be enough ventilation in the attic to allow the fan to do its job. I looked at a house where the entire family suffered from allergies. The attic contained both a whole-house fan and an air handling unit. The family used the air conditioning only during the hottest summer days; the rest of the time they used the whole-house attic fan.

When the fan was working, it increased the air pressure in the attic. Because the attic had inadequate ventilation, air entered the leaky air conditioning sys-tem and blew back into the living spaces instead of blowing out of the house through the attic vents. The attic was full of allergenic dust that was stirred up by the air agitation and then moved with airflows back into the rooms below. If you have a whole-house fan, check with the manufacturer of the fan and attic vents to be sure you have adequate attic ventilation. Keep in mind that the unobstructed (free) area of a vent is always less than the area you see, because the opening area is reduced by louvers and screens.

VENTILATION VIBES

In one attic, excess rather than inadequate ventilation turned out to be an insidious culprit that nearly drove the owner mad. The first time I spoke with the man, I wondered if he was imagining things. He told me he hadn't slept for a week because vibrations in his right lung were keeping him awake at night. I was about to say I couldn't help him when I realized I was committing what I consider a professional sin: doubting the client. I decided I owed him at least a house visit, and we made an appointment.

As soon as I entered his home the man dragged me frantically from room to room, asking questions about fiberglass and furnishings. Was the furnace too close to the wall? Could fumes off-gassing from the walls in the newly built home be causing his problem? I kept reminding myself, "The client is right; the client is right."

Finally he unwound a little and I was able to ask him some questions. I discovered he had been living there only a month, and for the first three weeks he had slept peacefully. What had changed in that last week? Contractors had installed a new floor in the attic just before his insomnia began. He led me to the attic, and there I saw the beautiful new tongue-and-groove flooring. As he walked about and I stood motionless near the stairway, I could feel the vibrations from each footstep. I suddenly realized that adding the flooring had stiffened the attic floor structure, making it respond to pressure the way a diving board reacts after the diver jumps up and down. Technically speaking, it was behaving like a damped harmonic oscillator: the energy in each footstep bounced the floor, causing vibrations that then diminished rapidly in strength.

The large master bedroom where the man slept was directly beneath the new attic floor. Nailed to the attic floor joists at the top was the new floor, and at the bottom was the bedroom drywall ceiling. As the attic floor vibrated, so did the attached ceiling, which in consequence compressed and expanded the air in his bedroom, changing the pressure within. For some strange reason the man was able to detect these pressure changes, but only in his right lung. I tested my theory by very gently bouncing up and down in the attic while the man lay on his bed beneath. About 70 percent of the time he could feel the vibrations as I moved. I decided he wasn't crazy after all.

What was making the floor vibrate? The attic was so well ventilated that when the wind blew outside it changed the interior pressure in the attic. When the attic air pressure was greater than the air pressure in the bedroom below, the floor was pushed down. When the attic pressure was less, the floor was pushed up. In both cases the floor movement caused vibrations that were transmitted to the air in the bedroom. Before the new flooring was added, the attic structure had not been stiff enough to vibrate this way.

I told the man he could hire an acoustical engineer, but I recommended that he first see if putting weight in the middle of the attic floor would diminish the oscillations. Since he had just moved in, all his books were still in boxes. He carried these to the attic and piled them right above his bedroom. After that he slept like a baby.

ATTIC AIR HANDLING UNITS

A man with young children became concerned when the family's nanny began to feel respiratory distress a few weeks after moving into their air conditioned home. He found it curious that she was suddenly suffering from the same symptoms everyone in his family had been experiencing, and he called me to investigate. I found that the return system for the attic air conditioner's air handling unit consisted of a duct attached to the blower cabinet at one end and to the fabricated metal box at the other. The metal box sat on the attic floor, partially buried in loose fibrous insulation, directly above the return grille that held the filter, flush with the second-floor ceiling. From a ladder on the second floor, I opened the return grille and removed the filter. Then I saw a one-inch gap between the metal box and the top of the filter holder. The seal between the box and holder should have been airtight, but because it was not, the air conditioning return was sucking attic air (full of allergens) and loose insulation fibers into the system, which was circulating the contaminated air throughout the house. After the family made the return airtight, installed a media filter, cleaned the ducts and AHU, and HEPA vacuumed all the rugs and carpeting, their symptoms decreased.

I investigated a similar case in which a retired couple had installed air conditioning three years before. The husband's allergies had seriously increased ever since. The air handling unit was in the attic. In this case the installer had never even bothered to put in a duct to the filter holder, which again was in the second-floor ceiling. Instead, he just cut a large hole in the wood floor of the attic and secured the return duct to it, assuming that air would flow between the joists from the filter at one end of the attic to the return duct at the other end. Unfortunately a one-inch gap between the ceiling plaster and the bottoms of the joists (which were supposed to form the return duct) allowed unconditioned and unfiltered air from the entire attic floor structure to enter the system.

One more caution: if the air handling unit for your air conditioner is in your attic, be sure there is adequate ventilation to keep the attic as cool as possible. The warmer the attic, the more energy it takes to cool the air within the duct system. It is more cost effective to ventilate an attic than to cool down heated air. An attic exhaust fan can be installed to increase ventilation.

ATTIC MECHANICAL EQUIPMENT

I am starting to find furnaces in the attics of newer homes. Many of the problems with furnaces in basements will also occur when they are in the attics. For example, dust, attic air, or loose insulation fibers can enter the heating system through leaky ducts. One arrangement that I have seen only twice, but that seems particularly unsafe, is a furnace humidifier in an attic system. If the attic is cold enough, the water supply pipe could freeze and break, flooding the entire house. Even if the pipe only leaks, the water can wet uncovered insulation, creating conditions conducive to mold growth. Never install a furnace humidifier in an attic.

Another problem common to both attic air conditioning and heating equipment is inaccessibility. It is very hard to service and repair equipment when the attic has no flooring. Sometimes the door to an attic is so small that the service company may not be able to use its best technician because the person is too large. If you have attic mechanical equipment, be certain there is ready access to the attic, that there is safe flooring all around any equipment that needs to be serviced, and that lighting is adequate. For families with allergies or asthma, attic equipment should be isolated from the general attic space inside an insulated, ventilated, well-lit mechanical closet. This also makes it easier to maintain the equipment properly.

If you have air conditioning equipment in the attic, be sure there is an over-flow tray with a float cutoff switch under the air handling unit. A secondary drain from the overflow tray isn't a bad idea, either, because if the condensate tray leaks, water will go into the overflow rather than onto the ceiling below. If you do have an overflow tray in your attic, check it during the air conditioning season to be sure the drain line is functioning and that no water is accumulating in the tray. On more than one inspection, I have found attic overflow trays full of water and moldy debris.

LIVING IN ATTICS

While renovating their house, friends of ours turned the third-floor attic into a spacious master bedroom and bath. The bathroom ceiling sloped because it was under the roof gable. The plumber foolishly installed water pipes on top of the insulation close to the roof sheathing. After the renovation was complete, the couple went out of state for a vacation. Before they left, on a cold winter day, the husband tried to take a shower in his new bathroom. There was no water, and he assumed something was wrong with the plumbing. He showered in the old second-floor bathroom, and the couple left for their long weekend.

While they were away the frozen pipes in the new bathroom burst and water cascaded down to all the rooms below. Fortunately they had asked a neighbor to check the house, and the flood was discovered before the interior was completely destroyed. When I saw the house, most of the floors had buckled, the walls were sodden, and a few of the plaster ceilings had collapsed. The insurance paid for the damage, but all the hard work and planning that had gone into the renovation was lost.

If you have pipes in your attic (or on the top floor of your house), be certain they are not on the cold side of the insulation. If you turn on a faucet in the winter and no water comes out, be warned! This means water has frozen in the pipes, and they might burst. (You can minimize the chance of bursting by allowing faucets to trickle.) And if you have any type of piping containing water in the attic and then decide to increase your attic ventilation, it's extremely important that you install insulation in a way that allows heat from the house to keep the pipes warm. It's not enough to insulate the pipes themselves, because insulation doesn't *create* heat, it only slows down heat loss.

If you own an older home with finished rooms under a sloped roof, there may be insulation under the floor in that top level. If large gaps exist between the floorboards, air will flow over the insulation to enter the room. This air can contain irritants that affect people with allergies or asthma. If this is the case in your home, you can either seal the cracks or install a new layer of solid wood or vinyl flooring (but not wall-to-wall carpeting!). Allergens can also come from closets or bureaus built in under the eaves, because they may be open to dusty construction cavities. If you have a built-in dresser under the eaves, pull out a drawer and look inside. The space should be enclosed and you should not be able to see rafters or attic insulation.

Even if attics aren't finished, they are sometimes used as living space. For example, sometimes people put a carpet down on an attic floor and let the children play there. This is a poor idea because of the irritants that can collect in attic dust. In one home, the attic dust was potentially lethal. I had almost finished the inspection when I went up into the attic. Most of the house had been well maintained, and up to that point in the inspection the buyer had been pleased with the condition of the property. As we ascended the attic stairs, I could see a rug on the floor and toys scattered about. The children had poked holes in the sloped plaster ceiling as they played. I could see the wood lath and rafter insulation through the ceiling gaps.

I thought the insulation looked odd, and bits of it seemed to be ground into the rug. I feared the worst. I opened the eaves closet and looked up at the rafter cavity with a mirror and a flashlight. I was astonished to find the cavity stuffed with asbestos pipe insulation. The seller was a plumber, and he must have used the rafter bays to "store" the insulation he had removed from old heat pipes. At that point my buyer walked away from the attic and the deal.

In this situation the owner knowingly brought the asbestos into the attic. Another type of insulation, called vermiculite, was installed by other people who didn't know it contained asbestos, though less than 1 percent. This insulation, sold in bags, all came from the same mine in Libby, Montana. Fortunately, it is rare. Finally, in some older homes loose, fibrous asbestos insulation was installed between the ceiling joists in attics. This is another reason attics should not be considered habitable spaces. If you choose to have asbestos-containing insulation in your home removed, you must have it done properly by professionals.

ATTIC STORAGE

Whether finished or unfinished, an attic provides a dry place to store family albums, clothing, seasonal decorations, old dishes, extra bedding, and furniture. Keep in mind, though, that attic dust can be very allergenic and irritating. In older homes with balloon framing this situation can be even worse, because dust from inside wall cavities finds its way to the attic. (In balloon framing, the stud bays are open from the basement to the attic, so an airflow system driven by convection can occur inside the walls. If the basement is moldy, the spores can flow up the wall cavities and into the attic air, settling into the attic dust.) Whether you have balloon framing or not, if you plan to store possessions in an attic, be sure to minimize airflows at the framing or around pipe chases. Last, an attic used for storage should have a securely attached plywood or plank floor, not only to make cleaning easier and prevent someone from tripping or even falling through the ceiling below, but also because if there is fibrous insulation and no floor, stored goods can become contaminated with dust containing fibers.

RECOMMENDATIONS

PESTS

- Replace old attic insulation if it smells. If there is evidence of mouse infestation, clean the attic structure and spray paint it to make dust adhere to the wood surfaces.
- If your attic is full of guano, consult a certified industrial hygienist and consider sending some of the droppings to a lab to find out whether they contain *Histoplasma capsulatum*.
- At the exterior of your house, be alert for openings in gutters or around soffits that might let pests get in. Make sure gable-end louver vents have screens.

AIRFLOWS AND HEAT LOSS

- Minimize ice damming by preventing heat loss from the house into the attic, but do not cover recessed fixtures with insulation unless the manufacturer allows it.
- Have insulated covers installed over the openings at the attic stairs and over the top of a whole-house fan to prevent heat loss to the attic in the winter.
- Have a kill switch for a whole-house fan installed in the attic to prevent accidental winter operation.
- Make sure the connections in an attic return and supply system are airtight.

EQUIPMENT

- Be sure mechanical equipment in the attic has adequate flooring, lighting, and access.
- Don't install a furnace humidifier in an attic.
- Install an overflow tray with a float switch beneath an attic air conditioner AHU.

DUST AND ALLERGENS

- Don't use your attic for storage unless it has a securely attached plywood or plank floor.
- Keep in mind that gaps between attic floorboards, as well as closets and drawers built into the eaves, can be sources of allergens.
- If you have allergies or asthma, always wear a fine-particle mask when you go into your attic.
- Change your clothes after spending time in a dusty attic.
- Keep attics as clean and dust-free as possible.
- Remove or cover goods stored in the attic while a new roof is being installed.

MISCELLANEOUS

- Whenever possible, avoid placing water-carrying pipes in unheated attic spaces. Insulate the pipes so they will be less likely to freeze.
- When soffit or ridge vents are installed, be sure adequate openings are cut above or below the vents.
- Periodically monitor your attic for leaks, pest infestation, moisture condensation, and other problems.

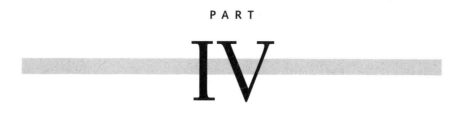

PART

IV

Clean It Up—Inside and Out

Renovation and New Construction

Your family grows, you decide to work from home, your new hobby requires a studio—any number of life changes can mean your current home is no longer large enough or arranged in the right way to meet your needs. In these circumstances, should you renovate or move to a different house? Although some people seem to pick up and move at the drop of a hat, most choose moving as a last resort. Moving can be fun and exciting, but it can also be a nightmare.

Many, many prospective buyers have asked me to do home inspections. Their anxiety over the details and deadlines involved in buying a house (the search, the offer, the negotiating, the inspection, the mortgage, the lawyers, the closing) keeps them awake and spoils their appetites. For people with allergies, asthma, or chemical sensitivities, the search for a new home is particularly complicated. And that's just the buying side. When people sell a home, they have to clean it up and prepare it for the market and try to get used to strangers marching through making comments about the furniture and the decor. And what happens if you're allergic to dogs and a prospective buyer's pooch leaves dander on your couch? But even though real estate transactions can be traumatic, particularly when air quality is an issue, people continue to buy, sell, and move. And whether you stay in your current home or move to a new one, renovation will probably enter your life along the way. The intent of this chapter is not to offer general construction advice but to provide some

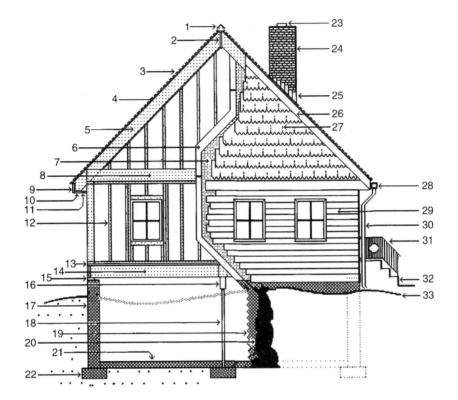

FIGURE 13.1. Schematic diagram of a single story house from the gable end. The basement is below grade.

1. Ridge vent	12. Stud	23. Chimney flue
2. Ridge pole	13. Subfloor	24. Brick chimney
3. Roof shingles	14. Floor joist	25. Chimney flashing
4. Roof sheathing	15. Sill	26. Rake trim board
5. Roof rafter	16. Main beam	27. Wood shakes
6. Wall sheathing	17. Foundation wall	28. Gutter
7. Housewrap	18. Beam support	29. Clapboards
8. Ceiling joist	19. Foundation	30. Downspout
9. Fascia board	20. Tar waterproofing	31. Handrail
10. Soffit board	21. Concrete floor	32. Stoop
11. Soffit vent	22. Footing	33. Grade

guidance for families with allergies, asthma, and chemical sensitivities who must deal with renovation and construction.

When I'm not inspecting houses, I'm just another homeowner—a prospective buyer and seller. In the more than twenty years we've been married, my wife and I have moved four times. I really dreaded our last move. We were living in a small house we had thoroughly restored, and everything was to our liking. We had even designed the kitchen with the counters and cabinets higher than usual, since we are a tall family. There were only two serious problems with the house. First, we were running out of room. Our children were getting older and bigger, and they were beginning to have their own social lives. One night my wife and I were sitting at the kitchen table, moaning about feeling more and more squeezed in our own home. At first our two children had their bedrooms and we had the rest of the house. Now we felt as if we had our bedroom and they had the rest of the house. We live in a city, and unfortunately there was no space on the lot for an addition. The second problem was that the house had a forced hot-air heating system, which was beginning to bother me as well as our son, who has asthma. It was time to move again.

We found a large Victorian that was "dehabilitated." The floors were covered with old wall-to-wall carpeting and glued-on cork tiles. Some of the original architectural details had been plastered over. The kitchen and bathrooms were old, and the pink walls in some of the rooms made me see red. I was dreading what faced us, but the house had forced hot-water heat and the space we needed, and it was in our price range. We made an offer and were rebuffed. We tried one last time, making an offer that was to expire at 11:00 P.M. At 10:00 the broker called to let us know the sellers were probably not going to agree to our terms. We were so relieved that my wife and I celebrated with champagne and looked forward to yet another lovely (though crowded) winter in our little jewel of a house. As we were going to bed at 10:50, the phone rang again. "Congratulations," the broker said. "We reduced our commission, and the sellers accepted your offer. You have a new home."

Before we moved in, we updated the kitchen and baths, had the carpeting removed and the floors sanded, tore down some false partition walls, and painted the rooms. After we moved in there was still much to do on both the interior and the exterior. We took care of leaky pipes, broken sash cords, and wiring that was not professionally installed. We graded the land around the house and landscaped the yard. We had to cut away bushes that were growing right up against the house, and we hired people to trim trees whose branches extended over not only our roof but the neighbors'. We had a mason fix many of the loose and cracked stones on the back patio. The asphalt driveway was crumbling, so that too needed to be redone.

One of the first things we did after we moved into the house in November was hire a contractor to replace the roof shingles on the turret. At the same time, the workers repaired and replaced some of the decayed soffit. As soon as the work started I began coughing, and I continued to cough after they had finished the job, packed up, and left. Even though the work was on the exterior, the hammering must have disturbed ancient moldy dust in the soffit, wall cavities, and attic. The dust could then enter the house air through electrical outlets, openings in window jambs, and other obscure pathways like pipe chases, abandoned ducts, and gaps in the flooring. Clearly, some fine particulates in the disturbed dust were irritating my lungs. Two weeks after the workers left we HEPA vacuumed surfaces and aired out the house, and at last I stopped coughing.

RENOVATION DUST

Dust is an inevitable by-product of renovation, including painting, so people with allergies and asthma need to stay away from the areas where the work is taking place. When large-scale projects such as moving walls, installing windows, laying new floors, and adding rooms are being done, I recommend that people with asthma or allergies not stay in the house at all. If that's not possible, or if the job is not extensive, the work area can be physically isolated from the rest of the house. Remove personal possessions, hang heavy plastic over the doorways, and operate a fan on exhaust in a window in the work area. (The fan will make the air pressure lower in that particular room than in the adjacent rooms, creating negative air pressure, so air from the rest of the house will go into the room being renovated rather than vice versa.) Buy your own drop cloths, because those owned by the contractor can be contaminated with all sorts of irritants (dander, mold, and dust from plaster or lead paint), either from other jobs or from a contaminated storage area. If you have a hot-air heating system or central air conditioning, be certain the registers and grilles in the space are covered while dusty work is under way. If heat supplies and returns have to be functioning in the work area, install high-quality filter materials over them.

Even if the construction area is isolated, workers should still be cautious as they come and go through the house, particularly if the residents have significant allergies. Dust from their clothing and shoes or from construction materials carried in and out can easily settle into rugs and furniture. If workers must move through other rooms in the house, lay down heavy construction paper to make a path. If necessary, isolate openings to other rooms with hanging plastic. If possible, have soiled materials removed through a window or a basement door. Walls and floors that are being dismantled can contain irritating dust and mold. Lightly spraying water on structures that are to be demolished or on surfaces being swept can reduce dust aerosol.

Sometimes I see dogs on construction sites because workers have brought their pets with them. If you are renovating your home or building a new one and are allergic to dogs, be sure none of the workers keeps a beloved pet inside for company. A few weeks of daily bombardment with dog dander are enough to thoroughly contaminate any hot-air system.

At the end of the day, don't let the workers clean up with a shop vacuum, since this may defeat all your precautions. The filtration in every shop vacuum I have ever seen is inadequate, and dust is spewed into the air. If possible, use a HEPA vacuum for all cleaning, and be sure the work area is kept sealed until the cleaning is complete. When the job is done, damp wipe all the surfaces.

Even smaller projects such as hanging a picture, putting in a new electrical outlet, or installing a phone line can kick up irritating dust. When you drill a hole to hang a picture, for example, plaster dust is released into the air and onto carpeting. If the wall is covered with horsehair plaster and you are allergic to horses, you may have a problem. Whenever I disturb the plaster in my older home, I have someone operate a HEPA vacuum while I work. Changing a sash cord in an old double-hung window isn't major renovation work, but you are still disturbing potentially irritating dust, so be cautious. If you have asthma or are bothered by dust, wear an N95 NIOSH double-strapped fine-particle mask when you or others are doing even minor renovation work in your home. Take your mask off after, not before, you change your dirty clothing.

PAINT
Lead Paint

By now most people know the dangers of lead paint, but I still hear stories about homeowners who are doing their own renovations. When repainting walls, they often sand old paint that has lead in it. One young couple was putting their house on the market because their second child had just been born and they needed a larger home. The listing real estate agent suggested they could increase the home's appeal by repainting the interior. While they were still living in the house, they began preparing the walls and woodwork for painting. Being diligent people, they thoroughly sanded all the surfaces in the century-old house. The house was marketed before all the painting was completed, and the couple received a strong offer more quickly than they had anticipated.

The buyers hired me to do their prepurchase inspection, which does not include testing for lead paint. For efficiency and convenience, the buyers arranged for a lead paint inspector and me to be at the property at the same time. While I was testing electrical outlets in the new baby's room, I noticed a look of great concern on the lead inspector's face. A few minutes later he took the buyers and me outside for a consultation. He said the levels of lead in the house were the highest he had ever seen—that even the infant's blankets and teddy bear were contaminated with unsafe levels of lead dust. He told us he was going to warn the seller to evacuate his family immediately.

Lead paint is an oil-based paint that consists of pigment, linseed oil, and solvent. The lead is in the pigment, a very finely ground white powder. The obvious purpose of pigment is to color the paint, but a less obvious yet even more important function is to hide the color of the surface below. One reason lead pigment was so widely used in the past is that it has extremely high hiding power. The linseed oil formed a binder for the powdered pigment, and the solvent thinned the pigment and binder so the mixture could be applied with a brush. After the oil paint was spread the solvent evaporated, leaving a viscous film of pigment and binder. Oxygen from the air combined with linseed oil in the coating so that it thickened, eventually "drying" to a hard plastic film. A very small amount of a sweet-tasting chemical called lead acetate (referred to as "sugar of lead") was sometimes added to paint to speed the drying. Paint containing lead pigment is *not* sweet, but people have believed this because of the chemical additive's common name.

Paint that peels from a surface usually comes off in large chips, and children get lead poisoning by eating those chips. I also believe that children can be poisoned by ingesting lead paint dust. Paint that is weathered or sanded from a surface consists of either microscopic pigment particles or barely visible dust particles. Children who touch the surfaces and lick their hands can easily ingest particles that settle on surfaces or mix with other types of dust in carpeting.

If you want to do cosmetic work in an older home, don't start sanding the painted surfaces (or let anyone else do so) before you've had the paint tested for lead. Most hardware stores sell inexpensive lead paint test kits, or you can hire a lead paint inspector to do the test for you. If lead paint is found, it should be mitigated by a professional according to whatever local, state, and federal regulations apply.

A house should always be thoroughly cleaned (including the furnace and ducts of a hot-air heating system) after lead paint is removed. One woman had many environmental concerns about her new home. Because she had young children, she wanted to be sure it was as clean and safe as possible before she moved in. The house had already been deleaded, and she asked me for some IAQ suggestions. I removed the grille from the floor return duct. The area just inside the duct had been thoroughly vacuumed, but when I looked deeper with a mirror and a flashlight, I could see a mat of dust over an inch thick. I took a sample and sent it to a lab for lead analysis. The laboratory found over 1,100 parts per million (ppm) of lead in the dust. I told the woman to postpone moving in until her furnace and ducts were professionally cleaned and the whole house completely HEPA vacuumed afterward.

The soil around a home whose exterior has been repeatedly scraped and then repainted with lead paint can have high lead concentrations, although a great deal of the lead in soil is residue from leaded gasoline. (According to EPA federal guidelines, over 400 ppm lead in bare play area soil is considered a hazard.) If you live in an older home and have young children or plan to have a flower or vegetable garden, it's a good idea to have the soil around the house tested for lead. Because of the potential risks, children should not play in soil within three feet of an older house.

If children play in a highly contaminated area, the dirt that sticks to their shoes can be carried into the house, particularly if they wear sneakers with waffle-patterned soles. The lead contamination can then be distributed into rugs or wall-to-wall carpeting, and they will continue to be exposed when they play there. Lead dust that is introduced into carpeting from contaminated soil, used drop cloths, or sanded surfaces can *never* be completely removed, no matter how frequently the carpet is washed or vacuumed. The carpet will continue to be a hazard for children for years to come. As I have mentioned before, vinyl and wood floors are preferable to carpeting because smooth surfaces are easier to keep dust-free.

If you suspect your carpeting is contaminated with lead, take a vacuum sample of the dust and have it tested. If the concentration of lead is high and the lab notes a health risk, get rid of the carpet as soon as possible, using the same caution as for the removal of any lead-contaminated material.

Oil and Latex Paint

Oil paints today are made with ingredients similar to those in lead paint except that the pigments contain no lead. About half the volume of liquid in a can of oil paint is a volatile thinner, and indoor spaces where painting is being done fill with solvent fumes as the thinner evaporates. Some states have banned oil paints. Today most paint is water-based (latex) paint and doesn't contain significant amounts of linseed oil or solvents. Latex paint does contain pigment and binder, but instead of being mixed with the water as a continuous fluid, the pigment and binder are suspended in the water. The binder is dispersed as microscopic oily droplets, similar to the way butterfat is distributed throughout cream. This type of mixture is called an emulsion. In latex paint, chemicals must be added to keep the oily droplets from coalescing and to prevent microbiological decay during storage in the can. (If old latex paint smells sour, don't use it; there is biological growth.) Other chemicals are added to control flow (viscosity).

After latex paint is applied to a surface, the water and some of the other added volatile chemicals evaporate. Once the water is gone, all the oily droplets coalesce to form a coherent paint film. The pigment particles that were suspended in the water end up stuck in the film. Latex paint on a brush and in freshly applied films can be removed with water because the droplets are still dispersible. But once the water evaporates and the droplets coalesce, water cannot remove the paint because water and oil are immiscible (they do not mix).

The air in a room may be irritating while the water and chemicals added to latex paint are evaporating. Although the risk is far less than with oil-based paint, those with chemical sensitivity should still be cautious about entering a space that has recently been painted. If off-gassing from oil or latex paint bothers you, check in your hardware store for the most environmentally safe paint. John Bower's *The Healthy House* also lists environmentally safe paints (see the resource guide at the end of this book).

When water-based paint first appeared on the market, it was called latex because the white binder emulsion resembled latex "milk," a natural product gathered from rubber trees much as sap is collected from maple trees to make syrup. As far as I know, latex paint never really contained latex from rubber trees. Today "latex paint" is a generic term for water-based paint. The paint is completely synthetic, and the binder is generally acrylic or vinyl. People with latex allergies should of course check with the paint manufacturer to be certain the emulsion is latex-free, but it is highly unlikely that any room painted with a newer, water-based paint would present a latex risk, despite the moniker.

Paint Stripping and Painting

Homeowners doing renovation projects often remove nonlead paint. People with asthma probably shouldn't strip paint without checking with their physicians, and everyone should use respiratory protection. Regardless of the method, removing paint entails exposure to dust or fumes. Scraping off paint fills the air with dust. Chemicals evaporate into the air. I read a newspaper story about one man who was using a chemical stripper to remove paint at the bottom of a closed stairway. The vapors from this particular paint stripper are denser than air, and because he was in a small, enclosed space, the vapors eventually displaced the air where he was working. The fumes contained the solvent methylene chloride, which in high concentrations is a "narcotic" and makes people drowsy. The man probably became confused, and according to the newspaper account he died from asphyxiation.

What is the purpose of having a toxic solvent in paint strippers? Paint, if properly applied, sticks like glue. Paint films on wood are particularly tenacious because the surface is uneven. To get an idea of the microscopic appearance of a wood surface, imagine cutting across a bundle of straws, exposing the numerous parallel channels (see chapter 1). Paint flows into the channels, and when it hardens it fits like a key in a lock. The solvent methylene chloride has a unique property: it diffuses into the paint film and makes it swell, just as water makes a dry sponge swell. Once the film swells it becomes flexible, and its bond with the wood is weakened. The paint can then be more easily scraped off the surface.

A few brave souls strip paint with heat guns, which produce toxic smoke as the paint is thermally decomposed. The film becomes less viscous and therefore softer as its temperature rises. There is thus a temptation to overheat the film and speed up removal. Unfortunately this produces more smoke (in part owing to thermal decomposition) and increases the likelihood of fire. Many buildings, including historical ones, have burned to the ground because of impatient or careless use of heat guns.

Most people sand a surface to prepare it for repainting rather than stripping off the old paint layers. This creates dust that should be contained. The area should also be sealed and ventilated during painting. Be sure to allow time for any volatile compounds to evaporate from the paint film before moving back into the space.

ASBESTOS

Asbestos is another hazardous substance that can be disturbed during renovation. One family installing new flooring in a finished basement used a floor sander to remove the old glued-on floor tiles. The tiles contained asbestos, and the collection bag allowed contaminated dust to escape into the air. The house dust became so filled with asbestos fibers that family members developed skin rashes. The entire house had to be professionally cleaned.

Asbestos is a mineral fiber that for years was frequently used in construction materials because of the benefits it offered. For example, asbestos fibers are not combustible, so they were used for fireproofing. Pressed together and shaped into cylinders, asbestos fibers were used as pipe insulation. Asbestos fibers reinforced floor tiles, joint compound, and exterior roof and wall shingles. Asbestos (like horsehair) was added to skim plaster both to strengthen the material and to give it texture.

Plaster containing asbestos is a composite, a mixture of two or more materials that has properties superior to those of the separate ingredients alone. For example, paper falls apart when immersed in water, and thin layers of wax are brittle, yet if you soak heavy paper in wax the composite can be used as a container for liquid (milk, for example), and it doesn't break when bent. Particle board, another composite, is made of "sawdust" and glue. Concrete and asbestos also form a composite. Concrete less than an inch thick breaks easily. If enough asbestos fibers are added, however, the concrete is strong even when thin, and the resulting composite can be formed into roof tiles or siding shingles.

One buyer asked me to inspect a recently renovated million-plus-dollar home on a large lot. She warned me the seller had disclosed that the fifty-year-old roofing shingles were made of an asbestos-cement composite. I looked at the roof from the ground with binoculars, and the shingles seemed to be in satisfactory condition. But when I went up to the attic bedroom and looked out the dormer window onto the roof surface, I could see that the shingles had worn thin and that white tufts of asbestos were sticking up where the concrete had weathered away.

It then occurred to me that the asbestos eroding from the surface of the roof might be ending up in the gutter and then in the soil around the house. I put a ladder up at the front of the house near a porch gutter. The debris in the gutter, normally leaves, was in this case white. The buyer took a sample of the gutter debris and sent it to a lab for analysis; it was 25 percent asbestos. Where the gutters were overflowing at another spot, soil was splashing up against the side of the house. I took a sample of the caked-on dirt, and that too was sent for analysis. The sample contained 10 percent asbestos. Needless to say, mitigation of the roof and soil was needed, and it proved costly.

Finding Asbestos

Inhaling asbestos fibers can cause a rare type of chest cancer called mesothelioma years after exposure. There are three common mineral forms of asbestos fibers: amosite, chrysotile, and crocidolite. Fortunately chrysotile, the form of the mineral most widely used in the United States, is generally considered the least carcinogenic. Still, asbestos is a dangerous substance and must be handled carefully and eliminated when possible by a trained professional.

If your house has or ever has had asbestos roof shingles, there could be a significant level of asbestos in the soil around the building. Asbestos-cement siding shingles generally are not as much of a concern because they are not subject to erosion by rain as roof shingles are. Asbestos siding can also be painted, which helps prevent release of fibers.

If you want to remove asbestos siding, the same care must be exercised as in removing roof shingles containing asbestos. I was inspecting the outside of one house and noticed numerous light-colored chips on top of the soil. I suspected they might be broken bits of asbestos-cement shingles. I asked the owner about them, and she proudly replied that it had cost her only $500 to have a neighbor remove all her siding. Unfortunately the neighbor obviously was not qualified to do the work. If you suspect you have asbestos outside or inside your home, have the materials or soil tested. If you know you have asbestos on your roof or heat pipes and furnace, do not remove it yourself. Always have asbestos professionally mitigated, or you and your family could be breathing in the fibers for years to come.

Your basement is a good place to start if you are looking for asbestos. I have seen many homes with older hot-air heating systems (the "octopuses" I referred to in chapter 10) that had the furnaces and ducts wrapped in asbestos insulation. We had asbestos pipe insulation in our own Victorian, and the day after the closing I hired a professional mitigator to remove all of it. I prefer removal to encapsulation (or wrapping), because the cost of the two options is about the same and, more important, if any repair to the heating system or pipes is needed, asbestos-containing materials will still have to be disturbed even if they are encapsulated.

I have my own asbestos story to share. Before I started my inspection career, our daughter attended a parent-run preschool in the basement of a church. We had monthly parent meetings, and at one such gathering, the coordinator was about to end the discussion when she asked if anyone had any other concerns. Relieved that the meeting was about to close, I leaned back in my chair and looked up at the ceiling high above. I noticed that the insulation on the many steam pipes was falling off. When I stood up and walked over to the toy shelf directly beneath the falling insulation, I was horrified to see clumps of what looked like asbestos-containing material covering the toys.

I spoke up and said, "Yes, I think I have a concern."

The next day, classes were suspended while a representative from an asbestos mitigation company came to investigate. He told us to close off the room and have the entire space professionally mitigated. Toys were cleaned or thrown out; the carpet was discarded. It was two weeks before the children were allowed back into the room.

Asbestos can be found in areas other than the basement. I inspected one house that had been foreclosed and then abandoned. The roof had been leaking, and the moisture had caused widespread damage to the ceilings and walls—a shame, because the hundred-year-old house had many wonderful architectural details. The oak and maple floors were littered with chips of plaster from the walls. When the house was built, a skim coat of plaster textured with asbestos had been applied to make the walls look like stone. Though determining the presence of asbestos is not a part of a prepurchase home inspection, I could see small tufts at the edges of the broken chips. The buyer sent samples of the chips to a lab for testing, and the results were positive. Before selling the foreclosed home, the bank was forced to do a very costly cleanup.

UREA FORMALDEHYDE FOAM INSULATION

Older houses were not built with wall-cavity insulation. During the energy crisis in the 1970s, however, many people decided to insulate. Some added siding that had insulating qualities, but more commonly they blew or pumped insulating materials into the wall cavities from either inside or outside the building.

Several types of insulation can be installed in this way, including loose fiberglass, cellulose (finely shredded newspaper containing about 20 percent fire retardant), and urea formaldehyde foam insulation (UFFI). This foam is no longer used, for reasons discussed below, though another kind is now available. A foam consists of a composite of a gas and either a liquid or a solid. Some common foams found in our homes include whipped cream, shaving cream, foam pillows, and computer mouse pads. Breads and cakes are also foams that have been cooked into place.

Insulation is meant to slow heat loss from the interior of the house during the heating season and reduce heat gain from the exterior during the cooling season. Heat can travel in three ways: convection, conduction, and radiation. *Convection* is heat transfer in a fluid (like air or water) by bulk movements of the fluid, owing to differences in density. For example, if you put your finger in a glass of cold water, the water around your finger is heated and rises by convection. (Remember that when a fluid such as air or water warms, it becomes less dense and rises.) In heat loss by *conduction,* energy is transferred from particle to particle by collision. If you heat the end of a metal rod in a fire, for example, eventually you will have to let go of it, because the heat will travel up the rod by conduction. Some metals conduct heat better than others: copper is a good conductor, but iron is not. Because steel is made from iron, good stainless steel pots have copper bottoms to help spread the heat more evenly. Similarly, rock is a better conductor of heat than wood. This is why granite feels cold when you touch it (it is conducting the heat away from your hand) and wood feels warmer (less heat is lost through conduction, so you "feel" your own hand's warmth). If you pick up an empty foam cup, it too feels warm, because the material doesn't conduct heat well.

When heat is lost through *radiation,* infrared energy (one form of heat) goes into space away from the heat source, in the same way that visible light is broadcast from a lamp. If a red-hot object sits in a room, it gives off light and heat. Both travel in straight lines and can be reflected by a mirror. If you stand in front of a fireplace you can feel the heat of the fire; but if people stand in front of you, you cannot, because they are absorbing the radiant heat (you are standing in their "infrared shadow"). In the late afternoon of a hot summer day in the city, even though the air may be cooling as evening approaches, it always feels hotter than it actually is, because the asphalt and the building surfaces are reradiating the heat energy they absorbed from the sun during the day.

UFFI and other insulating materials slow down heat loss mostly by reducing convection and radiation. The rate of heat loss by conduction depends on the density of a material, or how much matter there is in a given space. The greater the density, the more rapid the heat loss by conduction. Foams are not very dense and thus do not conduct heat well. Air is also not very dense. You might think that by filling a wall cavity with anything other than air you are in fact increasing heat loss by conduction, and you might be right. When the wall bays are filled with insulation, more heat may be lost by conduction, but there is minimal heat loss by convection because the air can't move around freely anymore; and the reduction of heat loss by convection is much greater than the increase of heat loss by conduction. Because any insulation fills a wall cavity, heat loss by infiltration and exfiltration is also reduced.

Now, what's the problem with UFFI? This insulating foam, which was used in the United States only from 1970 to 1979, was made from two liquids that were mixed on site (at the home). If the liquids were not mixed in the correct proportions, formaldehyde was released from the foam into the house. High levels of formaldehyde can make some people ill, but most homes insulated with this foam are now considered safe because the off-gassing has ceased. If you have UFFI in your home, you can obtain a testing kit to measure the concentration of formaldehyde in the air. (UFFI doesn't release much formaldehyde in dry air, so the test is accurate only if the relative humidity is greater than 50 percent. The windows in the house must be kept closed to minimize dilution by infiltration and exfiltration.) I am not concerned about UFFI if the levels of formaldehyde are low. There may be market implications, however. For example, in Massachusetts sellers have to disclose the presence of this insulation. In the 1980s the selling price of some homes was reduced by as much as 30 percent if UFFI was present.

If you find a foam material in your home, don't automatically assume it's UFFI. Many homeowners use foams from an aerosol can to insulate smaller spaces and cavities. When these foams set, they form a very tough, elastic solid. UFFI, on the other hand, crumbles to dust when it is touched, and a piece of it feels almost as light as air. (Be careful about inhaling UFFI dust; I heard about one case where individuals became sensitized.)

HOME OFFICES

Many major renovations are undertaken to add office space to a home. More and more people are working from their homes, and the old "study" is evolving into a professional office with desks, swivel chairs, copiers, fax machines, computers, and the like. People with allergies, asthma, and chemical sensitivities must be cautious when working in home offices, because the furniture and office machines may cause problems.

I encourage people to increase the ventilation in a home office. Install exhausts for office machines or place them in their own well-ventilated space. Photocopiers may emit small amounts of ozone (a potentially irritating gas) and styrene (another irritating volatile organic compound and a potential carcinogen). Photocopying uses a very high voltage on an electric wire. If you have ever smelled a shirt hung outside to dry on a sunny day, you can recognize the odor of ozone. Even though the smell may remind us of stepping out in the fresh air, excess levels of ozone are associated with air pollution.

Another odor that comes from copiers is produced by heated plastic. An image being transferred to paper initially consists of powdered black ink that contains carbon, plastic, iron particles, and small amounts of solvents. The paper then passes through a fuser, which is a very hot wire in a glass tube. When the ink absorbs the radiant heat from the fuser it melts, causing the plastic to stick to the paper. Some of the heated plastic thermally decomposes, producing by-products that can be irritating. Plastics in computers, video monitors, and cables also off-gas irritants or even smell like mold!

If you find your home office is bothering you, or if you are chemically sensitive, I recommend you purchase metal office furniture and avoid fabric chairs (see chapter 2). Remember that dust mite allergens can accumulate in the cushions of an office chair. A leather-covered chair is a good alternative.

OTHER CAUTIONS ABOUT ADDITIONS AND NEW CONSTRUCTION

On an inspection of a newly constructed house, I once overheard a buyer commenting to the real estate agent that she preferred not to live in a used home but wanted a new one instead. You may think you are avoiding allergens by purchasing a brand new house, but this may not be so. If you have asthma or allergies, you must use caution regardless of the age of the house. After all, if you aren't energetic about protecting yourself, who will be?

Whether you are building an addition to your home, living in a newly constructed house, or planning to build a home from the ground up, I have several pieces of advice to share.

It's always cheaper to build an addition over a crawl space than over a full basement, but don't be seduced (see chapters 8 and 9). If you must have a crawl space, be certain the floor is poured concrete. I don't recommend insulating between the floor joists with fiberglass, because of the numerous problems already described. Instead, the walls of the crawl space should be insulated with sheet foam (foil faced, a minimum of one inch thick or whatever is required by the building code in your locale). Preferably the crawl space should be open to a basement that is dehumidified in the summer and heated in the winter rather than disconnected from the basement and vented to the exterior. Check with your local building department on the use of sheet foam in basements.

When insulation is blown into walls, the air used pressurizes the wall cavities and disturbs all the dust at the same time. The air has to come out somewhere, and most of it exits to the exterior through the holes drilled in the siding. Some air can enter the living spaces, however, through electrical outlets, switch plates, and window gaps. If you are planning to have insulation blown into your home and are allergic to house dust, seal all gaps in interior walls and arrange to be out of the house during installation. When the installation is complete, you should HEPA vacuum your home and air it out well.

I discourage families with allergies or asthma from installing wall-to-wall carpeting in renovated or new spaces. I inspected one new house in which the installed carpeting was off-gassing so strongly it was difficult to spend time there. Most manufacturers recommend that people ventilate a house thoroughly after installing new wall-to-wall carpeting.

In earlier chapters I have mentioned many problems with wall-to-wall carpeting as well as other concerns that are relevant in new construction. I won't repeat all that information here, but I do want to discuss new homes with hot-air heat and central air conditioning. In every new house I inspect, I look into the ducts with a mirror and flashlight and find all sorts of debris: sawdust, drywall dust, pieces of wood, and even tools. On one inspection I found a doughnut bag with food and a coffee cup inside, and the duct was full of sawdust and plaster dust. I told the buyers to insist that the heating system and ducts be professionally cleaned (a costly effort) before they closed on the house. They asked me to reinspect the property shortly before the closing date, and I made a point of checking the duct where I had seen the doughnut. The duct looked cleaner, but when I removed the register and looked in with a mirror and flashlight, I could see that someone had cleaned only the end of the duct by inserting a vacuum into it. Now that old doughnut was even farther away, joined by a roll of duct tape. Even if people are just having floors sanded, I always recommend that hot-air heating systems and ductwork be sealed or protected by filters if possible, then thoroughly and professionally cleaned after the work is finished. When you purchase a new house, insist that the air conveyance system be as clean as the rest of the house.

I corresponded by e-mail with a woman in the Midwest who told me she had developed asthma and mold allergies after her home was flooded. She tried everything she could think of to clean up the house, but her efforts seemed futile. She decided to sell the house and build a new one that would be environmentally safer for her. She hoped she would be able to stay in the old home until the new house was ready, but the air made her feel so ill that she began to sleep in her car.

She wanted to have baseboard heat in the new house instead of hot-air heat, but the builder persuaded her to install a forced hot-air system with air conditioning. The new home was completed in the middle of the summer, and as soon as she moved in, she turned on the air conditioning. Within a few days her asthma symptoms increased. The air conditioning had been operating when the builders were working on the house, and I suspect the entire interior of the air handling unit became coated with construction dust that then got wet from condensation. She suffered for months and even considered moving again, but she ended up replacing the ducts and having the AHU professionally cleaned. All the fibrous lining material had to be replaced.

A home that has been flooded can be renovated, but any possible sources of concealed decay must be eliminated. One family purchased a home that had been extensively renovated after a serious flood. Many of the ceilings and walls had been replaced, and new bathrooms and a new kitchen had been installed. Unfortunately the warped maple flooring had been left in place, covered with wall-to-wall carpeting. After the renovation the husband, who worked on small carpentry projects in the basement, began to have trouble breathing. He was diagnosed with asthma and severe allergy to mold, and he was finding it increasingly hard to control his symptoms.

I found large clumps of very fine dust hanging in strings from the basement floor joists. Each clump was directly below a gap in the plank subflooring. When I looked at the dust samples with a microscope, I found they consisted of numerous *Penicillium* mold spores, decayed cellulose, bits of carpet padding, and insect fecal material. I suspect that after the flood, water was trapped between the subfloor and floor, and extensive decay and mold growth followed. Whenever anyone walked on the carpet above and the loose maple floor flexed, dust was forced out of the spaces between the subfloor and floor and into the basement air (though some of the dust stuck to the joists). After my visit the owner decided to look at the dust more closely. He did not wear a mask, and he touched the material directly. Within hours he was wheezing and had hives. He is planning to remove the carpeting and maple flooring. Before new hardwood flooring is installed, the moldy subfloor may also have to be replaced.

If you are sensitized, handle dust that may be contaminated only with the utmost care. If you have asthma or allergies and you are considering purchasing a home that has been renovated, be sure to find out if there has been any flooding.

Some construction materials can cause trouble for people with sensitivities. Although suppliers of paints and other building materials may claim their products are less irritating than others on the market, for chemically sensitive individuals any product can be threatening. Try to obtain a sample of the material before it is applied or installed, to see if you react to it. As I noted above, John Bower's *The Healthy House* is also an excellent source of information on building materials.

Surprisingly, one material you should check before it goes into your building is wood. In the basements of many new homes, I have found floor joists covered with mold. The surface of even pressure-treated wood (wood treated with copper arsenate to prevent decay caused by mold and insects) can support mold growth. The preservative protects the cellulose, but the sugars in the wood sap probably leach to the surface, allowing microorganisms to degrade it.

AIR-TO-AIR HEAT EXCHANGERS

To solve indoor air quality problems, some people have installed air-to-air heat exchangers. These devices bring in fresh outdoor air and exhaust stale indoor air. To save energy during the winter, heat from the exhaust air is used by the heat exchanger to warm cold incoming air; during the cooling season, incoming air is cooled by the outgoing air. Unfortunately, none of the devices I have seen were properly maintained or designed, and all were contaminated with mold growth. They had inefficient fiberglass filters and insulating liners with exposed fiberglass; the insulation in some of the units was soiled and stained from water that had condensed when humid air was cooled. If you purchase such a device, be sure it is equipped with 40 percent efficient media filters, that there is no exposed fibrous lining, and that all the interior components are accessible for cleaning. Change the filters and check the ducts twice a year.

RECOMMENDATIONS

RENOVATION

- During renovations, physically isolate areas under construction, cover or remove personal possessions, and create negative air pressure.
- Use clean drop cloths.
- Install filter material at hot-air registers.
- If possible, keep the heat or air conditioning turned off.
- To clean, use a HEPA vacuum.
- Keep out of the work areas. If you must enter, wear a fine-particle mask.
- Seal all gaps in exterior walls and arrange to be out of the house during installation of blown-in insulation. HEPA vacuum your home after the procedure has been completed.

ENVIRONMENTAL HAZARDS

- Have the paint in your home and the soil outside tested for lead. If you suspect or know that the soil around your home contains lead, do all you can to prevent dirt from coming into the house. Have your children take their shoes off at the door, for example. Ask your local health department for advice.
- Don't sand lead paint.
- Always have lead paint and asbestos professionally mitigated.
- If you suspect your home contains UFFI or other items that may emit formaldehyde, use a test kit (see the resource guide).

MISCELLANEOUS

- If you are selling your house and you have allergies, ask the listing broker to alert agents that prospective buyers should not bring pets with them.
- If you are chemically sensitive, install an exhaust system for home office copiers and printers, or place these machines in their own well-ventilated space.

14

Cleaning

In many of the homes I have described the rooms seemed spotless, yet people were experiencing indoor air quality problems. I make my living in part with my microscope, and when I examine dust, even from homes that look clean, I often see particulates that may be allergenic.

What can sensitized people do to keep their environments *really* clean? Earlier chapters dealt with specific areas of the house. This chapter is dedicated to the general relation between cleaning and IAQ concerns.

VACUUMING

One tenant had lived in her home comfortably for many years, but two years before she called me she had developed a persistent cough and frequent sinus infections. She thought something in the apartment might be causing her symptoms. She had vacuumed as well as she could, and she had even consulted a psychic (not a step I generally recommend!), who suggested cleaning the drains. Nothing seemed to make a difference, so when a similar apartment in the same complex became vacant, she was considering moving.

Before she made her final decision, she slept in the empty apartment for several days and was relieved to find that she didn't cough. She committed to the apartment and had new carpeting and a new refrigerator installed before moving in. Soon after she settled into her new home, her cough returned. She gave up the fight and temporarily moved in with her parents until she could figure out a solution.

Because the woman's allergist found she was allergic to dust mites and other common allergens, she asked me to see if I could find any sources. We decided it would be a good idea to check the level of dust mite allergens in her couch. The woman used her own vacuum cleaner to obtain a dust sample. By the time she had finished collecting the dust (about three minutes), she was coughing so violently that she ran to the bathroom and vomited. I went out on the front stoop and took a Burkard sample of the air at the vacuum exhaust; it was full of mold spores and dust mite fecal pellets. The concentration of dust mite allergens in the couch was almost 25 micrograms (mcg) per gram (g) of dust (above 10 mcg/g is considered a risk for asthma sufferers). Her vacuum cleaner may have been removing surface dirt from the couch, but it was also sucking up mite allergens and spewing them into the air.

We think of a vacuum cleaner as a machine that draws dirt in, but in fact it's pulling in air that contains the dirt. The air flowing into the machine has to flow out, and we hope the dirt and dust particles will remain behind in the vacuum bag. This usually doesn't happen with microscopic particles, however, because most vacuums are leaky. Particulates exit around seals and from within the vacuum bag itself. In addition, vacuuming vigorously with any type of equipment disturbs the carpet surface, releasing additional contaminants into the air.

Some vacuum cleaners have special filtration. I prefer a vacuum with a HEPA (high efficiency particulate arrestance) filter that is supposed to contain all large particles and at least 99.97 percent of the 0.3 micron particles suspended in the air moving through the machine. *I continue to recommend that those with allergies in the family use only a HEPA vacuum.* If you plan to purchase one of these machines, check *Consumer Reports* magazine for the latest evaluation of the various models. One client spent $800 on a low-quality vacuum that had an "optional HEPA" filter attachment, which she also purchased. The filter holder was secured to the vacuum by two plastic tabs that fit into holes much larger than the tabs. Most of the exhaust air blew unfiltered out of the openings around the tabs, completely defeating the purpose of the HEPA filter. If you do buy a HEPA vacuum, be sure the holder is airtight and that the filter is properly placed in its holder. Follow the manufacturer's recommendations for filter replacement. If you are very allergic to dust, wear an N95 NIOSH fine-particle mask to change the vacuum bag (outside the house), and be sure the inside of the compartment that holds the bag is clean. Avoid using a bagless vacuum; dumping the dust may create allergenic aerosol.

Another costly type of filtering vacuum cleaner uses water to trap the dust. I took an air sample at the exhaust of such a vacuum and found many aerosolized particulates. One scientist found that cat allergen from dander in house dust dissolved in the water and was then emitted back into the air as a finer aerosol than when it had entered. In addition, people don't always follow instructions for the proper use of these vacuums. The water is supposed to be emptied when the vacuuming is completed, but one man left the water with the dust in the vacuum, which he then stored in a closet. You can imagine what grew in this dusty reservoir!

Some people prefer to install a central vacuum system rather than using any type of portable vacuum cleaner. If you have a central system, be absolutely certain the exhaust vents to the exterior, not to the garage or basement. (The outside vent should be as close to the motor as possible. If the exhaust path is too long, back-pressure might reduce the airflow.) If dust collects around the unit, your blower probably has a leak.

How often should you vacuum? I recommend cleaning floors and stuffed furniture with a HEPA vacuum at least once a week. If you have a regular vacuum cleaner and you are very allergic to dust, wear an N95 NIOSH mask and air the house out after vacuuming. *Never* use a shop vacuum to clean up dust in your house, and *never* use an ordinary vacuum for moldy dust. And remember, allergens such as dander and mites in your carpet can never be completely removed by vacuuming. You may have to replace your carpet if the irritants prove too troublesome. If you have lead paint dust or asbestos fibers in your carpet, you may want to have the carpet removed by a professional. Testing for lead and asbestos is inexpensive, so when in doubt, take dust samples. (If you have to replace a carpet, always replace the pad and HEPA vacuum the floor first.)

CARPET CLEANING

Some advocates of carpeting claim that carpet acts as a dust "filter," storing dust until it can be vacuumed up. They maintain that rooms with carpeting have fewer airborne particulates than comparable rooms with hardwood flooring. In the sense that it accumulates dust, carpeting does act as a filter, but like all filters, anytime the surface is disturbed some dust is released. And unlike carpeting, when most filters are dirty they are replaced.

In all the hundreds of homes I have inspected, I always find that the air in spaces with wall-to-wall carpeting contains higher concentrations of particulates than the air in spaces with hardwood, vinyl, or ceramic flooring. Even the air within the same home contains fewer particulates in rooms without rugs or carpets. (To support claims of benefit, I suppose that if the same amount of dust was placed in two experimental rooms, one with carpet and one without, and the air was sampled while a small room fan was operating, you would find less aerosol in the room with the carpet because the fibers trap some of the dust. However, such an experiment would not be representative of an actual home where the fibers themselves are regularly disturbed and not just the air.)

Though dust accumulations can be diminished by vacuuming thoroughly twice a week with a HEPA vacuum cleaner, keep in mind that (as one quantitative study showed) even after dozens of passes dust can never be completely removed from a carpet. (Try this experiment if you want to prove this to yourself, but if you are allergic to the dust, wear a mask: In the dark with a flashlight on the floor, briskly rub a carpet with your hand to observe the dust cloud; vacuum the surface as you normally would and rub again.) The thicker the carpet, the greater its capacity for collecting dust.

When your carpet gets dirty enough to wash, be sure to hire a trained professional. When people wash their own carpeting using rental equipment, the machine may either apply too much water or be unable to remove enough water. If carpets stay damp, bacteria and fungi will start to grow. Many people have told me that their carpets remained damp for more than a day after being washed and smelled for a while longer. Even though the smell may go away, I believe that the carpet forever after contains biological organisms and their byproducts that will be aerosolized with every footstep.

DUSTING AND WIPING SURFACES

Just as walking on a contaminated carpet releases irritants into the air, cleaning surfaces with a feather duster only resuspends the settled dust. Dust should be either HEPA vacuumed or wiped up with a clean, slightly damp cloth. You may recall the story about the dirty sponge and the conference table in chapter 6, and throughout the book I've stressed the problems excess moisture can cause. The lesson here is don't use a dirty dustcloth and avoid soaking surfaces.

Recent studies have demonstrated that regular application of antiseptic sprays drastically reduces the level of viable mold spores and bacteria on surfaces. But in most cases this spraying is unnecessary; in fact it can introduce irritating fragrances and chemicals from the spray itself into the interior air. Trying to eliminate the background level of microorganisms that can settle on surfaces is futile, because wherever there are people, there is an endless supply of skin scales, and wherever there are skin scales, there are bacteria and yeast. And this doesn't even take into account the mold spores suspended in the air that infiltrates a home from the outside. To minimize the nutrients available for living organisms, just dust surfaces regularly. If an individual is sensitized to particular components in the dust (such as dust mite fecal material or mold spores), the source of the irritants should also be eliminated—otherwise allergens will continue to collect.

Some dust reservoirs are more important than others. The dust balls behind a bed's headboard may not have much impact on your life, but the dust near a hot-air register, computer fan, or refrigerator may become aerosolized and find its way to your lungs.

LAUNDROMATS AND DRY CLEANERS

If possible, it's probably a good idea to do your laundry at home if you have serious allergies. If you use a public laundromat, the dryer may contain residues of irritating detergent, fragrance, and fabric softener.

I find walking by a laundromat irritating because the dryer exhaust is always contaminated with laundry chemicals (I took an air sample at one dryer exhaust and collected numerous respirable detergent particulates). If people who are chemically sensitive live downwind from a laundromat or a dry cleaning establishment, or even in an apartment near a communal laundry area, the odors and particulates could affect them. (One client was so bothered by the detergents from the basement laundry that she bought an acceptable detergent for all four of the other families in the building.)

Dry cleaning makes use of a solvent, usually tetrachloroethylene (perchloroethylene, PCE). When you pick up a suit or a dress at the dry cleaners, the clothing usually retains a chemical smell from the residual PCE. If this bothers you, air out the clothing before bringing it into your home or hang it in a well-ventilated room. But remember to remove the plastic bags.

DANGEROUS MIXTURES

Ammonia and chlorine bleach should never be mixed because they form a poisonous, carcinogenic gas called chloramine. The labels on these products warn against this, but keep in mind that other cleaning products may also contain ammonia or bleach. For example, some scouring powders contain chlorine bleach, and some dishwashing liquids contain ammonialike compounds. Be careful about what you mix together. You may think of cleaning products as benign, but in fact they may be powerful chemicals. Follow label directions, believe the warnings, and use ventilation as needed.

One additional warning: If you have a swimming pool, be extremely careful to keep any bromine- or chlorine-containing biocides out of the house and away from any other chemicals. The fumes alone can be irritating, and the compounds themselves are dangerous. For example, if a chlorine-containing biocide comes in contact with some algicides (also used in pools) or other household chemicals, the mixture can burst into flames.

CLEANING COMPANIES

If you hire people to clean, be sure they use only *your* vacuum. If they use their own vacuum cleaner and it leaks, you can be certain that allergens from the last few houses they cleaned will be distributed into the air in your home.

I worked with one family whose allergy symptoms were increasing, particularly after their home was cleaned. I took Burkard air samples in the house and concluded there was cat dander in the carpets. The couple was astonished, because they had never owned a cat and the carpets were relatively new. I asked what type of vacuum they used, and they told me they hired people to clean. The cleaning company first vacuumed the neighbor's house, where a cat was happily shedding, then ran the vacuum in my clients' home, where it spewed out cat dander that rained down on all the carpets.

CLEANING AND PETS

We love our pets, and we like to hold them and pet them. If you have allergies to pet dander, wash your hands after touching an animal. Bathing dogs and cats helps wash off epidermal scales and allergens. (One family installed a Victorian tub on legs with a hand shower in the basement to hose down their golden retrievers.) Use a HEPA vacuum in your home, for just as we shed skin scales, pets shed dander. Remember my caution in chapter 3: four-legged pets are living dust mops and will spread any contamination they pick up throughout the spaces where they roam. For example, if your carpeting is contaminated, the fur of the dog that lies on it will be too.

If your pet has a special blanket to sleep on, wash it frequently. Don't use expensive quilts or thick pillows for pet mattresses, because they can be reservoirs for mites and other allergens and can never be completely cleaned. Keep in mind that the fewer cushioned and fleecy surfaces you have, the fewer the reservoirs for dander. Don't let shedding animals lie on stuffed furniture.

Having a pet means that dander will spread throughout the house, but try to keep a dog or cat out of the bedrooms to minimize the spread of irritants. If you make the difficult decision to give away a pet or if your pet dies, remember that the dander will remain in the house dust on and in everything, including beds, furniture, rugs, radiators, ducts, and refrigerators. Don't expect any lessening of symptoms until all the house dust is eliminated.

WAGING THE WAR

Most people get upset when they see critters scurrying around their homes. It's creepy to see a mouse run out from under a kitchen cabinet, ants crawling in the pantry, or a bee swooping across the room. Often the first thought is to rush out to the hardware store for a can of pesticide. I encourage you to resist this impulse. I don't recommend using spray pesticides indoors, because these chemicals can have toxic effects on the hunter as well as the hunted. In addition, poisoned mice can die inside walls and cause odors. It's much better to use ant baits (which keep the chemical fairly well contained), depend on a rolled-up newspaper (no toxic effects there!), or buy a sticky mousetrap.

Having to fight microscopic life forms can turn people into fanatics. To deal with dust mites, they sometimes do the equivalent of bombing an entire village to capture one soldier. They eliminate their curtains, shades, carpets, bedding, and stuffed furniture. They buy new mattresses and pillows. They add acaricide powders (which kill mites) to all fleecy surfaces. Such steps are indiscriminate. Instead, people should focus on the source of the allergens and start by cleaning thoroughly and using allergen-control mattress and pillow covers (see the recommendations at the end of chapter 3). For example, if a mattress and pillows are the sources of dust mite allergens, the allergens will also be in the dust in the curtains. Encasing the mattress and pillows will eliminate the source, then the curtains can be washed and rehung. The curtains should never again be a problem.

There are two kinds of acaricide powders: one type has benzyl benzoate and acts only on dust mites; another type contains borate, which affects most insects. Both chemicals are relatively nontoxic but can be expensive. In addition, the fragrance in benzoate products can be bothersome. Most important, neither the borate nor the benzoate affects existing mite allergens. These chemicals are toxic only to living mites and have no effect on irritants in the mite fecal pellets. Thus you might not see any improvement in symptoms after using such miticides.

Confirming a dust mite infestation is the first step. I encourage people who are allergic to dust mites to buy a sampling bag from a laboratory and send samples of the dust from their mattress, pillows, and carpeting off for testing. This analysis may be more costly than acaricide powders, but minimum testing may be worth the expense, depending on the size of your home, how many people live there, how much wall-to-wall carpeting you have, and how much of your furniture has fleecy surfaces. Identifying the source of allergens is vital in a successful campaign.

If you live alone and have only one bed, for example, you may prefer to buy the allergen-control mattress and pillow covers. If you have a larger family and also own many pieces of stuffed furniture, the testing will help you find out whether you have dust mites, where they may be, and the concentration of allergens. The more knowledge you have, the better armed you are for the fight.

"DRY" STEAM

For mitigating allergens, I recommend steam (water vapor) instead of typical carpet cleaning equipment, which uses only hot water. When rugs and carpets are cleaned with hot water (often referred to as "steam cleaning") the material takes longer to dry out, creating a better opportunity for mold and bacterial growth. In addition, when the hot water hits the room-temperature carpet, the water cools and is thus less effective in destroying organisms. Steam (pure water vapor), on the other hand, is an outstanding method for killing dust mites, spiders, carpet beetles, and fleas—anything that may be living in a carpet.

In the past few years, home versions of steam-generating cleaning equipment have come on the market. These machines look like vacuum cleaners, are relatively easy to use, and produce steam that can kill all insects and denature (destroy) allergens in furniture and carpets.

It may be less expensive to steam your carpets than to replace them. One of my clients was having increased difficulty with his allergies when he was at home. He had three floors of wall-to-wall carpeting that I found was full of dust mites. He decided to steam the carpeting, and because this type of cleaning is slow-going, he spent several weekends working at it. In the end, it was worth the effort. He told me that after all the carpets had been steamed his symptoms abated. Steam cleaning allowed another homeowner who was highly allergic to cats to reoccupy her home after tenants moved out leaving cat dander behind.

Why is steam so much more effective than hot water? This question leads into a brief discussion of the three phases of matter: solid, liquid, and gas. Water is the liquid form of H_2O; in its solid state, H_2O is ice; in its gaseous state, it is water vapor. When ice becomes liquid water, the H_2O is undergoing a phase change from one state of matter to another. The same is true when H_2O changes from liquid to vapor during evaporation or boiling. A solid is in a more ordered state than a liquid, and a liquid is more ordered than vapor. ("Ordered" indicates the way the molecules are arranged. In a solid the molecules are all spatially arranged in a pattern, often crystalline. In a liquid and a gas they are constantly moving and rotating. In a gas the molecules are about ten times as far apart as in a liquid or a solid.)

Energy is always required to change matter from an ordered to a less ordered phase. Heat energy changes ice to liquid water and liquid water to vapor. It takes about five times as much energy to change a cup of water to vapor as to heat the cup of cold water to the boiling point. As the water changes to vapor at the boiling point ($212°F$ or $100°C$), both the liquid and the steam are at the same temperature, but the steam contains far more stored energy. Steam thus has much more heat energy to lose than does hot water at the boiling point.

Suppose you steam a sofa. When the steam hits the room-temperature surface, a very small amount of it condenses to liquid; the phase change releases the stored energy and heats the couch material to the boiling point of water. In addition, the steam continues to flow, and because it is a gas it penetrates the cushioning, raising the temperature of the stuffing.

If applied long enough, steam not only kills insects but also denatures many allergens. I tested the effectiveness of steam by applying it for different lengths of time to certain sections of a mattress that contained about 40 mcg/g of dust mite allergens. I divided the mattress surface into four parts. One part was my control; this section I did not steam. I steamed a second part for ten minutes, the third part for twenty, and the last part for thirty. A few hours later, after the mattress dried, I took dust samples from all four sections. I found what I had expected: the longer the steam application, the lower the concentration of allergens. In another experiment, steam reduced dog allergen in a cushion from over 30 mcg/g to less than 1 mcg/g. (Unfortunately, you must experiment to find out how long to steam any particular item.)

There are several cautions to keep in mind when using a steam machine. First, be sure the high temperature will not harm the material you are steaming. Steam can damage the finish on a hardwood floor, for example, so area rugs should be steamed outside or above the floor. Second, steam can cause burns, so be very careful while using a steam machine and follow closely the manufacturer's directions for maintenance and use. Last, don't let moisture build up in an enclosed space, because this can cause paint to peel.

AIR PURIFIERS

There are two major categories of air pollutants: particles, and gases or vapors. An air purifier with a HEPA filter is designed to eliminate particles (particulates). Air purifiers with charcoal are intended to adsorb formaldehyde and solvent and other vapors from the air. The hitch, though, is that the "filtering" ability of the charcoal doesn't last very long. At one point I borrowed a "used" portable air purifier with both a HEPA filter and a charcoal filter. After I turned it on, my entire office smelled of cigars. So much for charcoal!

People with asthma and their families spend money unnecessarily (in my opinion) on air purifiers, in the belief that they can clean the air. Air purifiers are unlikely to be useful, however, unless the sources of the allergens or irritants are removed. In other words, it is impossible to "clean" air when it is repeatedly contaminated by either surface dust or dust from rugs, pillows, mattresses, quilts, and the like. Conversely, dust in a home with few or no allergens is not as serious a concern.

I have seen people place $400 air purifiers in every bedroom. Some of these machines have blowers that exhaust high-velocity air out along the floor. In homes with contaminated carpets, the air stream disturbs the irritants in the carpets and makes them airborne. In several homes, I have sampled the air with the blowers off and with the blowers on, and at least initially I always found higher levels of particulates with the blowers on.

In the bedroom of one child with asthma, I started coughing as soon as I entered. An air purifier was operating. I turned it off and left the room. I returned twenty minutes later and had no trouble breathing. I wasn't surprised to see that a sample of the carpet dust I sent off for analysis contained 20 mcg/g of mite allergens.

No matter what manufacturers claim, spending money on expensive equipment designed to make your air healthier is a waste until you reduce your exposure to allergens in your indoor environment. If you do plan to buy an air purifier, eliminate allergen sources first, and then buy only an air cleaner with a HEPA filter.

CLEANING OURSELVES

Some of my clients with serious allergies report having symptoms when they are near certain people. People who have pets, for example, carry dander on their clothing and in their hair. People who sleep on pillows contaminated with dust mite allergens can carry mite fecal pellets in their hair. In chapter 1, I talked about yeast that causes eczema and dandruff as well as asthma symptoms. Good old-fashioned soap has biocidal properties, and the longer you keep soap on your body, the more effective it is in killing bacteria and yeast. If you soap yourself thoroughly in the shower with the water off and wait a minute before you rinse, the soap will have a chance to do its work. (Just keep soap off the bottom of your feet so you don't slip.)

While we're on the subject, hair collects allergens and can be a source of irritants long after exposure. For example, on most typical nonwinter days, mold spores and pollen grains are in the air. If you go outside your hair will accumulate these particulates, and when you disturb your hair allergens can become airborne. If you are particularly sensitive, your allergy symptoms may increase. When you put your head on a pillow, your hair is around your face. It's a good idea to shampoo your hair after you've spent time outside in the pollen or mold season (fallen leaves can be moldy), or after you've been in moldy spaces or spent time with pets. Don't go to bed with wet hair, because mold may grow in a damp pillow. If you don't like washing your hair so often, wear a hat when you're near irritants.

RECOMMENDATIONS

VACUUMING AND DUSTING

- If you suspect the dust in your furniture or in your rugs or carpeting is contaminated, purchase a sample bag from a laboratory and return it for analysis of its contents.
- Use a HEPA vacuum. Change the bag outdoors and be sure the inner compartment is clean.
- If you have a central vacuuming system, be sure it vents to the exterior.
- If necessary, wear an N95 NIOSH fine-particle mask when vacuuming or dusting.

CHEMICALS AND CLEANING PRODUCTS

- Limit your use of products that have fragrances.
- If you are chemically sensitive, don't live downwind from a commercial laundry or dry-cleaning establishment.

- Check labels on cleaning products to avoid mixing chemicals that may react adversely with one another. Never mix ammonia with bleach.
- Store pool chemicals safely, preferably not in the house.
- Limit the use of pesticides indoors.

STEAM

- Use dry steam to reduce allergens and insect pests in furniture and carpeting.
- Don't use a steamer to clean area rugs on hardwood floors. Lift the rugs or steam them outside instead.
- Spot test fabrics and carpeting first to be sure they will not be damaged by steam.

MISCELLANEOUS

- If you hire people to vacuum your home, make sure they use your equipment, not theirs.
- Have your rugs and wall-to-wall carpeting professionally cleaned.
- If you rent your house to someone, be clear about restrictions on pets and smoking.
- Take advantage of the biocidal properties of soap.

CHAPTER

15

Exterior and Garage

Outside the house there are fungal spores, pollen, pests, and pesticides, and any or all them can find their way in. This chapter describes how your care and maintenance (or lack thereof) of outside areas can affect your indoor air quality. It's impossible to separate your home from its environment, but if you understand how problems evolve, you can reduce the flow of contaminants from the exterior to the interior.

For example, one family asked me to find out how mice were getting into their home. The basement was littered with exterior debris like the forest floor and sprinkled with the shells of sunflower seeds from the backyard bird feeder. The family never realized that at the back of the house there was a gap of about an inch between the sheathing and the foundation sill (the wood resting on the foundation). The previous owner had attempted to stop up the opening with fiberglass, but the rodents carrying in their pilfered seeds bypassed this obstacle with ease.

The lesson here is to avoid having spaces between the top of the foundation and the sill and not to leave other foundation holes open. For example, if you've had an oil pipe removed, fill the opening with mortar. Don't use fiberglass insulation to fill holes, or rodents and other pests may move in. If you can't easily see the sill or look under the edge of the siding, check the perimeter of the foundation very carefully with a mirror and a flashlight. Also be sure to check for openings around windows.

TERMITES

Termites are worrisome pests because they can cause structural damage. The treatments used to combat these insects can also impair indoor air quality. It's important to avoid pesticides whenever possible, and to do so you will want to minimize the chance of a termite infestation by understanding what termites are and how they live.

Termites can be found in most states; in Massachusetts, for example, termites affect up to 20 percent of homes. The common termite lives several feet under the surface of the ground. A subterranean termite colony includes workers, soldiers to protect them, and a queen to lay eggs. Some colonies consist of several connected underground nests.

Termites travel concealed in dark spaces or in tubes called "shelter tubes" or "mud tubes," about 0.25 inch (6 millimeters) wide, which they construct from sand and a secretion that serves as glue. Shelter tubes protect termites from predators such as ants. You will always find sand inside termite-damaged wood. Shelter tubes can be found inside or outside wood or rising up from cracks in foundation floors or walls. They are often found on stockade fences when the pickets are set in soil (untreated wood should never be buried). When wood beams or joists are heavily infested with termites, you may see tubes hanging down from the structure. The longest tube I ever saw ran up a foundation wall from the floor to the ceiling, and the widest was about 3 inches (7.6 centimeters).

Worker termites destroy wood by chewing it, but it is the protozoa (microscopic single-celled animals) in their guts that supply the cellulase enzymes to digest the cellulose from the chewed-up wood. Termites are drawn to wet, mold-decayed wood, and fungus ingested along with wood fibers provides them with necessary nutrients. Some mold volatile organic compounds (MVOC) may function like insect pheromones, attracting the termites. It may be small comfort to those who find termites in their homes, but it's worth noting that workers are commuters. They live in the soil and travel back and forth to your home to destroy it (though Formosan termites, recent invaders in the South, nest inside walls). Traffic inside shelter tubes can resemble rush hour on a freeway. Worker termites are about 0.18 inch (5 millimeters) long, but you will probably never see one crawling about, because they are as shy as they are completely defenseless. Workers are soft, move slowly, and have no claws or stingers for protection. They look like a grain of rice with two antennae and six tiny legs. The soldier termites that protect them are much more formidable, and are about 0.3 inch (8 millimeters) long and have large mandibles. If you break open a mud tube, the soldiers rush to the opening to defend the workers.

Untreated wood in direct contact with soil invites termites. Wood house trim, basement window sills, wooden steps, and even wooden fences should not be in direct contact with the dirt. If you have a woodpile in your yard sitting directly on the ground, this too may welcome termites, particularly if the wood is decayed. Even wood chip mulch can attract termites. Termites are small, but in large numbers they pose a serious threat to your home because they hollow out beams, joists, and studs from the inside. They usually leave behind the outer layer of structural wood, but by the time the pests have finished their meal the remaining material may be no thicker than a coat of paint. One home inspector described a time he vigorously "probed" the main beam of a house to show the buyers how decayed it was. For the sake of drama he bashed the beam with a hammer, and he was horrified when the entire bottom splintered open, spewing live termites onto the broker and his buyers.

Treatment

Whenever live termites are found in a house during a home inspection, treatment is recommended. For decades, treatment has consisted of creating a chemical envelope around the foundation. The chemical is injected into the soil at very high pressure, and the soil bearing the pesticide creates a barrier against termite intrusion. To prevent termites from entering the foundation wall on the inside, pesticide is often also injected into the soil beneath the basement floor through holes drilled about every 18 inches (46 centimeters) into the concrete at the perimeter. If a nest is under the middle of a basement floor in a home, perimeter treatment alone may not be effective. In this case the pest control operator will probably suggest injecting additional chemical.

Although thousands of homes are treated safely for termites every year, problems can occur. First, all the chemicals used are toxic. Chlordane, for example, is one of the many pesticides that in the past was used to combat termites. The soil around and under many "slab on grade" houses was treated preventively with chlordane. In some homes with heat ducts in or below the concrete slab, people became ill because vapors from the soil diffused into the ducts. Chlordane has been banned, but many homes have lingering effects, since this chemical, a chlorinated hydrocarbon, persists for decades. For example, after digging in the soil around the foundation of a house that had been treated with chlordane fifteen years earlier, I could smell the chemical on my hands.

In some homes with dirt crawl spaces, pesticides were "broadcast sprayed" onto the soil and wooden floor structure because that was easier than crawling under and injecting it into the dirt (see chapter 8). When chemicals are applied in this way, a great deal of surface area is exposed and soaked. The pesticide evaporates slowly for years, and the vapors saturate the air in the crawl space. Unfortunately the air pressure in most crawl spaces, particularly in the winter, is higher than that in the rest of the house, because air exfiltrates at the upper levels of a home and infiltrates at the lower levels, and contaminated air flows into the living areas. I have been in homes with crawl spaces that had been treated with chlordane where the basement or even the entire house reeked of termiticide. If you have a dirt crawl space that you suspect contains chlordane, I recommend having the soil tested by a lab; you may have to remove soil and install a concrete floor. If the wood structure was broadcast sprayed with a toxic, volatile, persistent pesticide such as chlordane, even the wood may have to be replaced or sealed.

Pesticides have to be carefully mixed and applied. In older homes with stone foundations, even properly applied pesticides can flow from the surrounding soil into the basement in the form of vapor. The pesticide may also enter the basement if an unexpectedly heavy rain occurs shortly after the chemical is injected into the soil. (Pesticide is applied as an emulsion: small drops of oil containing the chemical are dispersed in water. After the emulsion is pumped into the soil, the water eventually evaporates and the oil droplets spread out onto the soil particles and become immobile on their surfaces. But before the water dries out, the pesticide emulsion can be carried with rainwater into a leaky basement.)

I believe people can become chemically sensitive if exposed to pesticides, so I recommend my clients use one of the newer treatments. These consist of bait systems in which traps containing small amounts of relatively nontoxic chemicals are installed at the outside perimeter of a home just beneath the surface of the soil. These traps contain levels of chemicals that are primarily toxic only to termites. In theory the termites carry the chemicals back to the nest and poison it. As a termite preventive treatment, you can also have sodium octaborate solution (see recommendations at the end of chapter 1 and the resource guide at the end of the book) applied to the wood structure of a crawl space, back porch, or garage, or in locations where wood is close to grade. Since this chemical is soluble in water, its effectiveness is reduced on wood that is exposed to the weather.

"Do It Yourself" Disasters

Wasp sprays, ant sprays, and mothballs are readily available in supermarkets and hardware stores. All those ads about mothballs and insect sprays give us the impression that these chemicals affect only bugs, but that's not so. In one case a woman sprinkled an entire box of moth crystals into the soil of a crawl space under her front porch. Air flowed from beneath the porch and infiltrated the basement, and from there it rose into the rooms of her house, carrying pesticide vapors throughout the living spaces. She felt she was becoming ill from the fumes, so she hired an inept handyman to clean out the crawl space. He ended up burying more of the moth crystals than he removed, and the vapors continued to infiltrate. Eventually she became chemically sensitive, sold the house, and moved. Another homeowner decided to cure an insect infestation on his own by pouring quarts of chlordane all around the hollow-block foundation of his house. The young couple that later purchased the man's home became so ill they had to sell.

One family called a pest control company because they saw a carpenter ant in the kitchen. Instead of ants, the pest control operator found evidence of old termite activity, and he recommended treatment. It just happened that on the day of the treatment the city had temporarily shut off the water to the street for pipe repairs before the technician had finished diluting the pesticide. The PCO went ahead with the treatment anyway, inserting a long metal wand around the house at about two-foot intervals and pumping the incompletely diluted chemical into the soil.

The house had a leaky old stone foundation, and someone should have been on the inside to monitor the operation. Concentrated pesticide from the soil outside dribbled down the foundation walls and into the basement, and the family was forced to move out. To help eliminate the pesticide fumes, they operated their powerful whole house attic exhaust fan for two months in the vacant house. They left the door from the house to the basement open so that the air flow created by the fan would draw the pesticide fumes from the basement into the attic and outside. This wasn't a great idea, because it distributed the fumes throughout the house. To make things even worse, the depressurization of the basement air caused combustion gases full of carbon monoxide to backdraft from the furnace into the home.

Every time the family entered the house, no matter how briefly, they became nauseated and suffered headaches. The husband thought he could correct matters by "rinsing" the chemical from the soil with dishwashing detergent, and he poured dozens of bottles onto the ground between the shrubs and the foundation all around the house. Then he generously hosed the dirt. The bath didn't seem to help, so he purchased pumping equipment and injected hundreds of gallons of concentrated bleach into the soil in an attempt to destroy the pesticide. But the bleach combined with the soap and other materials in the soil to create a toxic cloud of gas, forcing people in surrounding homes to evacuate. Then the man called me. Should he inject hydrogen peroxide into the ground, he asked, to eliminate the chlorine bleach? I was astounded that he was willing to inject still more chemicals into the soil.

Pesticides are powerful chemicals. Don't apply them yourself if they require professional application, and be sure to use licensed, qualified workers.

THE NEIGHBORS' CHEMICALS

If you are buying a house and a member of the family is chemically sensitive, keep in mind that the appeal of the well-manicured lawn next door or the golf course down the street may be due in part to pesticides. It's worth a little research before committing yourself to the property. If a neighbor's pesticides bother you, at least plan to be away during application. If there is or used to be a gasoline station, a buried oil tank, or a light manufacturing operation next door, chemicals that were dumped or leaked from underground storage may have migrated through the soil to your property. This can result in toxic basement vapors.

If you are living in a house or are considering buying a house that you think has a peculiar chemical odor in the basement, again do your research and believe your nose. Don't let other people convince you that you're imagining things, and be suspicious of overpowering room deodorizers or potpourri. You can also purchase a test kit containing activated charcoal that adsorbs air contaminants (see the resource guide at the end of this book). The kit is left in the basement for several days and then returned to the lab for analysis.

Mold from neighboring properties can also be bothersome. For example, if you are downwind from a mulching facility or even a neighbor's compost pile, vast clouds of spores can be carried in air that intermittently flows toward your property and into your house.

VEGETATION

I peered under a deck during one home inspection and saw ivy growing up the foundation wall. One stalk caught my attention because it looked wider than the others. I crawled under for a closer look and pulled the growth off the foundation. Much to my surprise, I saw that termites had concealed their mud tube behind the stem.

I have seen much damage to buildings caused by trees and shrubs. In one house a tree branch moved by the wind rubbed a hole in the roof that allowed water in. Subsequent wall decay led to termite infestation. In several homes, leaves in contact with house trim deflected streams of rain onto the wood, causing rot. Dead leaves from overhanging branches can clog gutters, and a falling branch can damage a roof or skylight. Plants growing up against the siding also slow drying after rain. I always recommend that homeowners prevent plants from touching their homes and allow enough space for inspection between the foundation wall and all plantings.

People who are sensitized should be careful when handling vegetation. One of my clients developed hives while collecting cuttings from a shrub. Another man who didn't know he had allergies experienced asthma symptoms immediately after dumping a barrel of moldy leaves over a fence. If you are a gardener and have asthma or allergies, it's a good idea to wear an N95 NIOSH mask while handling plants or digging in dirt.

If you have allergies to certain plants, try to avoid growing them on your property. If you live in a wooded area, you may have to be particularly careful about poison ivy, which can cause a rash when touched and even when burned. Many people have had serious reactions when upwind neighbors burned poison ivy. Even if you aren't sensitive, avoid burning poison ivy, for someone who lives in your neighborhood may be vulnerable.

WATER, TOP TO BOTTOM
Chimneys, Roofs, and Gutters

If not properly channeled away from the walls and foundation, rainwater can fuel mold growth both inside and outside your home. Let's start at the top of a house and follow the various courses water may take as it makes its insidious attack on your property.

Here's a chimney story. One spring I received a call from a man who in the past year had had the exterior of his home repainted and new asphalt shingles installed over the old roof. After the first winter, stains and large water-filled blisters appeared in the paint film on the clapboards at the front of the house, between the windows of the two second-floor bathrooms. The contractor thought moisture from the bathrooms was the culprit, but the owner thought the contractor's poor prep work was at fault.

With a Tramex meter, I detected an elevated moisture content in the roof shingles above the stained and blistered area. I suspected that water might be getting in under the shingles from the chimney. Carrying a hose, I climbed onto the roof, where I found a large crack in the mortar cap at the top of the horizontal portion of the oversized chimney. The chimney was made of brick but coated with stucco. Shortly after I directed a small stream of water into the crack, moisture exited the stucco at about the middle of the vertical side of the chimney. I then knew that water was entering the crack, sneaking down the chimney between the brick and the stucco, and running unseen down the roof on top of the old shingles and beneath the new ones. Before the water reached the edge of the roof, it leaked behind the fascia board in the soffit and into the wall behind the clapboards. The moisture behind the clapboards passed through the wood as vapor and condensed behind the paint film. The accumulation of water had blistered the film. I advised the owners to install a leak-proof chimney rain cap, a metal or masonry cover supported about a foot above the flue opening.

If there had been flashing at the bottom of that chimney, it would have prevented the water from getting under the roofing. Chimney flashings are usually made of lead and are embedded in the mortar used to hold the bricks together. Normally the lead is bent flat against the brick, and each piece overlaps its neighbor. The chimney flashings at one home I inspected were bent upward and made the chimney look like a top hat. The tenants told me why. Apparently a raccoon had been living in the chimney on top of the damper of the unused fireplace. When the landlord discovered the animal, he covered the flue with metal mesh to prevent her from climbing down it. The raccoon was undeterred; in fact she was so infuriated that she bent all the chimney flashings up into the air in an effort to get back into her old home. She then found an area of the roof sheathing around the chimney that had decayed and made her new home inside the attic. Water leaked in around the hole and caused severe mold growth in the living room below.

When I'm inspecting homes, I always find that old chimneys with rain caps are in surprisingly good condition. If you have a chimney, it's a good idea to have a rain cap with an animal screen at the sides as well as proper lead flashing at the base.

Now let's move from the chimney to the roof. Obviously, if your roof is leaking you should have it repaired. Just because a roof is new, don't assume it can't leak. The old-style organic felt asphalt shingles lasted twenty to thirty years, but the newer fiberglass asphalt shingles may last only fifteen to twenty years. Premature failure of this newer material owing to manufacturing defects has led to roof replacements in as little as three years at thousands of homes. If you are replacing your roofing, try to get organic felt rather than fiberglass shingles, but check that the fire rating complies with your local building codes.

On rare occasions animals can chew holes in a roof or falling branches may cause damage. Never allow a branch to touch your roof, because movement caused by wind can lead to abrasion and holes. To check for leaks, look around your attic with a bright flashlight during a heavy rain. I also encourage people to have the branches of tall trees overhanging the roof cut away, because falling leaves and branches can clog or damage gutters.

Other roof problems can be created by design errors. In one home the family began to detect a powerful smell of mold after they completed a second-story addition, designed by a very inexperienced architect. All the roof water from the addition and from about a third of the original roof was channeled into a valley and from there to a narrow section of gutter, which did not have the capacity to handle it. Some of the overflow cascading down the wall entered the wall cavity through a gap around an exterior light fixture, and mold started to grow.

In homes without gutters, an adequate roof overhang is essential to keep water away from the walls and the foundation. Overhangs are particularly important for homes with hardboard siding and no gutters, because hardboard (a composite of sawdust and glue) absorbs moisture and swells at the cut ends and nailheads, leading to decay.

In one case, when a couple arrived to tour a house that was on the market, the owner was baking cookies. The price, location, and condition of the house, as well as the inviting smell, convinced the couple to buy it. During the home inspection, the different but still fragrant odor of plug-in floral air freshener welcomed them. The masking odor should have cautioned the home inspector (who had been referred by the broker selling the property), but in this case no warning flag went up. After the couple moved in and pulled the plug on the fragrance emitters, they noticed a strong odor of mildew. They eliminated all the old carpeting and gutted and remodeled the kitchen and bathrooms, but the odor persisted. Soon the husband, who had allergies, began to experience symptoms.

When the mildew smell became a stench, the couple called me. I walked around the outside of the house, and one of the first things I noticed was a large mushroom poking out of the hardboard siding on the shaded end of the building. I made several recommendations to improve the air quality inside the home, but my main concern was determining the condition of the concealed materials where the wall seemed to be decaying. I suggested the couple hire someone to conduct exploratory wall surgery.

A few months later I received a thank-you note telling me what had happened. There had been extensive decay at the back of the soaked hardboard siding, and mold had spread throughout the building paper between the siding and the sheathing. The couple ended up residing the house with vinyl. During the removal, the dumpster outside the house (containing all the decayed hardboard siding and building paper) smelled so strongly of mold that the couple could not remain in the house. In addition, several neighbors complained about the odor. Once the dumpster was removed and the house resided, the owners were able to move back into their "home sweet home."

Most homes should have gutters, which sit at the edge of the roof. If they are properly positioned and well maintained, gutters can prevent many moisture problems. They must be kept clean, and they must be wide enough to handle water flow, pitched correctly, and watertight at joints. There should also be adequate overhang at the edge of the roof (the soffit) so that if the gutters overflow, water will run directly to the ground from the roof edge rather than down the wall. The metal drip-edge flashing at the roof overhang must also be at the right angle to direct the water into the gutter and not behind it.

Despite their positive features, gutter systems are a common cause of water damage. Gutter joints and end caps often leak, causing paint to peel on wood trim below. Even the order in which the downspout sections are connected is important. Most of the water flowing within a downspout clings to its inside walls, and when the joints are reversed (the crimped "male" end of section facing up instead of down), a lot of water leaks out of the joints. In one home with reversed downspout joints, water leaked out and flowed down the outside of the downspout until its path was thwarted by the bracket that secured the downspout to the house wall. At that point the water was diverted toward the wall, where it flowed down the trim and soaked the wood. Termites moved in to complete the destruction.

Stand outside your house during a heavy rain and observe the gutters. If you see water dripping behind the gutters, leaking out of joints or end caps, or flowing on the outside of the downspouts, you have a problem. In my own house a gutter filled with leaves couldn't handle the water in a heavy storm, and the water streamed down the outside of the house to a kitchen window. Although the window was closed the storm window was open, and the space at the bottom of the window filled with water, which leaked through the walls and into the basement. It was quite a mess, and it all happened because I hadn't had a chance to clean out that gutter.

In another building the owner never cleaned the gutters. When they filled and overflowed, the curvature of the gutter channeled the overflowing water at one end into a stream that sprayed against the vertical corner trim boards of the house. Years of water entry caused severe concealed decay of the entire corner structure. Repairs entailed replacing the corner posts of the walls (a major structural repair) as well as large sections of the siding.

Cleaning gutters is a tiresome chore, and one that very few people do often enough, including me. Clogged gutters are far more likely if you have trees overhanging your home. Some people install gutter screens to keep out debris. In New England at least, these are rarely effective, because the ice that fills gutters every winter dislodges them. Those who are not physically active should hire someone to clean gutters. I know of two homeowners who broke their backs falling from ladders while doing this job.

When gutters aren't working properly for one reason or another, moisture problems are likely to follow. In one wood frame medical office I inspected, the gooseneck had fallen off so the downspout was not connected to the gutter. Water flowed out of the gutter down the side of the building and entered the wall cavity through a crack in a window sill. The entire wall cavity was full of mold. I was called to investigate because the examining room had to be abandoned after several patients complained of asthma symptoms.

Other Sources of Water Intrusion

Ice damming is another source of water damage at the outside of a house. As discussed in chapter 12, it is caused by heat loss from the attic through the roof. When wind drives rain against a house or when ice damming occurs, water can enter wall cavities through cracks in siding or gaps in trim. On many homes, wooden (or plastic) window and door frames and wood trim protrude from the siding of a building and can catch rainwater at the top edge. For this reason a window or door is often installed with a drip cap flashing that is supposed to shed water (the flashing is just an L-shaped piece of aluminum). If the flashing is sloped toward the building, however, it can channel water to the two ends of the flashing and from there into the joint between the vertical trim and siding and into the wall cavity. I have seen numerous new homes in which this condition has caused paint peeling and severe concealed decay and, in some cases, indoor mold odor. Be certain your drip caps are pitched

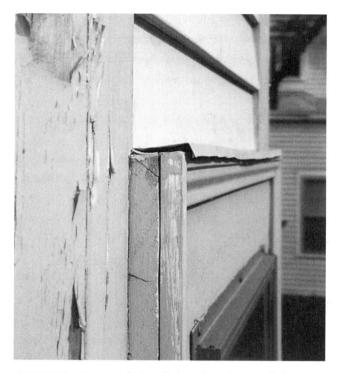

FIGURE 15.1. Improperly installed window drip cap flashing. The metal drip cap flashing on top of this window trim is bent up instead of down. As a result, rainwater that lands on the flashing is channeled to the side edges, where it soaks into and behind the trim, causing paint to peel. If this condition persists there will be concealed wall decay. To shed water, the flashing should slope downward all along its length.

correctly. Water should flow off the drip cap all along the edge, not just at the ends.

Water Dispersal

Properly working gutters and downspouts take the water to grade (to the ground), but it must still be directed away from the house to avoid basement moisture. If the soil outside the foundation is graded properly away from the building, then a downspout extension or a splash block should provide adequate dispersal. But if the grading is level or slopes toward the house, other measures must be taken (my advice is to regrade wherever possible). Many homeowners have the mistaken notion that if they can't see the water it isn't a problem. They simply bury the downspout in soil at the corner of the house without providing any piping to carry the water away, which often results in excessive foundation moisture.

Many people install dry wells, which are usually nothing more than reservoirs in the ground filled with crushed stone, although plastic barrels with pipe fittings are also used. Water from the downspouts is conducted through a pipe beneath the soil surface into the excavated area or barrel. Dry wells work for a time, but ultimately they become clogged with fine organic and inorganic material and cease to function effectively. When water can no longer be dispersed below grade by the dry well, it backs up and ponds around the foundation, often causing a wet basement. I recommend that people use a subsurface dispersal system where the pipe end discharges to daylight; this way you can see water coming out. (Just don't direct the water to the sidewalk or to your neighbor's driveway!)

Some home designs are more prone to wet basements than others. For example, if the footprint of your house is U-shaped, the water from one side of each of the three roof gables may flow toward the interior of the U. If the grading is level, as it usually is, excessive moisture soaks into the soil. In such cases more extensive methods of water dispersal must be in place. These may include sloping the land away from the building or installing subsurface drains (either with or without dry wells), or even creating a deeply sloped concrete or paved patio. A subsurface drain consists of a pipe that conducts the water away from the downspout and foundation to an area where it will not cause problems for you or your neighbors. The pipe must be pitched so that water drains out by gravity flow, and the end should be open to the air, not buried.

On the Ground

If, despite your best efforts, you have a buildup of water on the ground around your foundation, what can you do to minimize basement moisture? Be sure your basement walls are as watertight as they can be. Have major cracks professionally evaluated and sealed. Do all you can to have your land graded away from the house. If the wood siding doesn't have several inches of clearance from the soil, you can dig a trench around the foundation, partially refill it with crushed stone, and hold back the soil on the other side of the trench with a retaining wall made of treated wood or masonry. Keep the trench narrow enough so that water from an overflowing gutter will fall to the ground beyond the retaining wall.

Sometimes when the land slopes toward the front or rear of the house this cannot be changed. What you can do is regrade an area around the house to create a swale or moat that will contain the water flow and channel it away from the foundation. In older homes where the soil is eroded at the stone foundation, it is almost impossible to prevent water from dribbling in around stones. One way to minimize this type of water intrusion is to excavate around the perimeter of a home about 12-18 inches (30-46 centimeters) down and about 30 inches (75 centimeters) out. The bottom of the trench should be sloped away from the foundation and smoothed. A waterproof membrane (a deflection skirt) installed at the bottom of the trench is folded up against the foundation and tarred to it. You can even put crushed stone or a perforated drainpipe buried in crushed stone inside the trench. A layer of soil and filter fabric can cover the trench. This arrangement prevents surface water from flowing directly down the foundation wall, and if the trench has perforated pipe, water can be carried away from the building downhill to a remote site.

In places with cold winters, trenches of this kind can be particularly useful. If you live in New England or anywhere else with severe winter conditions, you may have noticed that snow tends to melt on the ground near foundations because of the heat loss from the basement. In the middle of the cold months the ground elsewhere may be frozen several feet down from the surface and thus be impermeable to water. If water ponds at the side of the house owing to ice damming or a winter rain, it will seep into the warmer soil near the foundation and may leak into the basement. An underground membrane and trench system provides a barrier that will direct this water away from the house.

Even if you have proper grading and a subsurface drainage system, if you don't maintain the wells around the basement windows you may still get water in the basement. Always be sure that water from downspouts flows away from window wells and that the wells are clean and free of debris. The soil in the well should be several inches below the window, particularly if the sill is wood. I have seen many termite infestations begin in buried wooden trim around basement windows. If you don't mind plastic covers, you can install one over a window well to keep the rain out. But be careful to keep the space free of leaves and other materials that can degrade, or you may end up with a mold odor around the window, which can be carried by air infiltration into the basement. If you are really sick of maintaining window wells and having water enter the basement from a window, you can always raise the level of the lower masonry and install glass blocks. Check your local building code, though, to find out the minimum number of windows required in a basement.

BULKHEADS, DECKS, AND PORCHES

Bulkheads are another concern. Sometimes people use plywood doors and ordinary pine trim to construct a bulkhead (a projecting framework with a sloping door giving access to a basement stairway). These are prone to decay from moisture and insect infestation; I prefer metal bulkhead doors. It's also important to keep the stairs and the space at the bottom and beneath them free of leaves and other debris, because moisture accumulates in these areas, leading to decay and mold. I often see newer homes with metal bulkheads but no interior doors. Metal doors are open to airflows and even mice. A bulkhead should always have an airtight interior basement door.

You must have a gutter above a deck, or large amounts of water will pour from the roof onto the deck and from there splash up onto the siding or, worse, into the framing beneath a sliding door. Decks and porches can fall victim to decay from excessive moisture if they are sloped incorrectly or if the trim at the edge is level or pitched toward the porch.

Water isn't the only problem with decks and porches. Odors can result from a variety of situations. Don't have your dryer exhaust vent under the porch or deck, for example, because moisture will usually condense on the wood, causing decay and odors. Another source of powerful odors is pest infestations (mice and other rodents) in accessible fiberglass insulation under porches. The moldy pest odor in one home was so powerful in the crawl space under a porch that it was very noticeable in the house and made the owner feel ill. He thought the smell was strongest at the top of the second-floor stairs and was concerned about roof leaks. Instead it was coming through gaps in the exterior wall and rising on warm air currents.

ATTACHED GARAGES

I was inspecting a newly constructed town house in a three-unit building. To my amazement, the hot-air furnace for each of the condominiums was suspended from the ceiling of the underground garage, hanging in the middle of what I expected would be a twice daily "rush hour" cloud of carbon monoxide. As is generally the case, the filter access at each furnace was not airtight, so whenever the blower operated it would draw in garage fumes. I recommended building an accessible, airtight plenum around the furnace (with an intake for combustion air), but the buyers fled the deal for other reasons.

I worry about attached garages, particularly those with bedrooms over them. Don't leave your car running in an attached garage, because carbon monoxide can rise to rooms above. Starting a car inside an attached garage is probably one of the largest sources of low-level carbon monoxide in homes. I recommend that individuals who are sensitized to gasoline not park the car in an attached garage. If you must keep the car inside, start it only with the garage door open. Allow time for the garage to air out before closing the door, and if this isn't adequate, install an exhaust fan on a timer. To prevent airflows into adjacent rooms, the door from the garage to the house should be made airtight with gasket material, and there should be no openings in the garage ceiling, particularly if there is a bedroom above. (An airtight ceiling, required for most attached garages, will also prevent smoke from spreading if there is a fire.)

Many newer homes have the electrical panel in the garage. Occasionally the cables from the panel go through a large opening in the ceiling, providing a pathway for auto exhaust and gasoline fumes. If you keep equipment such as a lawn mower or a snow blower in the garage, be sure it's not leaking. If possible, don't store gasoline (or pesticides or fertilizers with pesticides) in an attached garage.

Storing anything in a garage can cause trouble. People sometimes keep garbage or old, moldy furniture in an attached garage, and odors can enter the house. If you have exposed fiberglass insulation in a garage, rodents small enough to get under the garage doors will move in. If you live in a climate with snowy winters and park your car inside, large chunks of snow often stick to the rear of the car wheel wells, melt, and cause puddles that spread and soak into the walls, leading to mold growth and plaster damage. If you notice this happening, try to minimize the amount of snow you bring in with the car. If snow melts on the garage floor, mop it up.

In many new town houses I inspect, the bottom level consists of a one-car garage and an adjacent office. The driveway often slopes down sharply from the street. This design begs for water problems. In one case the town house was built between two asphalt parking areas that sloped toward the property. All the drainage and roof water from several adjacent homes ran onto the pavement in front of the steep driveway and down into the garage. In one storm the owners had more than three feet of water in the garage and basement office.

Even with more level adjacent grading, these steep driveways can collect rainwater during heavy rains. And it's often an easy step for water to move from the garage into the office on that level, where it wets the carpet and creates conditions conducive to mold growth and mite infestation. If you are living in a town house with this condition, you can install a drain with a powerful sump pump at the bottom of the driveway. You might also consider getting rid of the basement office space, or at least replacing the wall-to-wall carpeting with ceramic or vinyl tile. (Avoid irritating glue!) A more drastic option is to change the garage into basement space by replacing the door with a foundation wall and filling in the driveway with dirt. Just be sure that the new lawn is graded away from the house for water control.

People think of an attached garage as an exterior space, but it's not. Air from the garage can flow into the living spaces, and people with allergies and asthma should carefully maintain the area.

RECOMMENDATIONS

PESTS AND PESTICIDES

- Be sure any fiberglass insulation is contained so there is no pest access.
- Don't allow untreated wood (including piles of firewood) to remain in contact with soil.
- Check your basement periodically for termite mud tubes.

- When pesticides are necessary, have them applied by a professional.
- When buying a home, believe your nose; take odors seriously. If your home has a lingering chemical smell, consider purchasing a test kit. If soil in your crawl space has a chemical odor, have it tested for pesticides.
- If you are constructing a home with a crawl space, consider using pressure-treated wood there, or treat the wood with borate to minimize the threat of termite infestation.

VEGETATION

- Do not allow trees or shrubs to touch any part of the house. Maintain about 18 inches (46 centimeters) of clearance between the house and plant growth wherever possible.
- Don't let tree branches extend over your gutters or roof.
- Don't burn poison ivy or oak.
- Keep debris out of window wells, and keep the soil level several inches (over 10 centimeters) below any wood.
- If you have allergies or asthma, it's a good idea to wear a fine-particle mask and gardening gloves when handling plants or digging in dirt.

WATER

- Inspect the attic, the basement, and the exterior of your house during a heavy rain to watch for leaks.
- Consider installing a rain cap with an animal screen at the top of your chimney.
- Check gutters and downspouts to be sure they don't leak.
- Keep your gutters clean.
- If you don't have gutters, be sure you have adequate roof overhang.
- If you have hardboard siding, keep it painted, and never let roof water flow over it.

- Make sure the soil around the house is graded away from the foundation.
- Be sure drip cap flashings on windows and doors are pitched correctly.
- Don't allow roof water to splash onto a deck.
- Wherever possible, use subsurface dispersal for roof water and install the pipe so that water discharges to daylight.
- If your house is on a hill, divert water away from the foundation with a swale.
- If moisture leaks through your basement walls after it rains, clean the gutters, extend the downspouts, correct the grading, and then, if all else fails, install a subsurface deflection skirt around the foundation.

BULKHEADS, DECKS, AND PORCHES

- Use metal bulkhead doors.
- Be sure a bulkhead has an airtight interior basement door.
- Install a gutter above a deck.
- Avoid accessible fiberglass insulation under porches.
- Don't vent a dryer exhaust beneath a deck or porch floor or into a garage.

ATTACHED GARAGE

- Make sure the door from the house to the attached garage is airtight.
- Don't store leaky vehicles or gasoline containers in an attached garage. If possible, keep the mower in a separate shed.
- Don't let the car idle in the garage, even if the overhead door is open.
- If you're chemically sensitive, don't park the car in the garage at all.

16

Away from Home

In this country we spend over 90 percent of our lives indoors. In many metropolitan areas, underground shopping concourses connect buildings that are blocks apart. When we can't walk underground or in a mall, we drive from place to place with the car windows rolled up and the air conditioning or heat turned on. We step out of our cars into underground parking garages. We get our exercise in indoor gyms, swim in indoor pools, and jog on indoor tracks. We play tennis in "bubbles."

Indoor air quality is a concern not only in our homes, but in all the enclosed spaces where we spend most of our lives. Many buildings have bioaerosol problems. If you are sensitized, you don't have to spend much time inside to start having symptoms. Laundromats, fabric stores, hardware stores, furniture and carpet showrooms, shoe stores, and car dealerships can cause difficulties, mostly owing to off-gassing of volatile organic compounds and to fragrances and pesticides. This chapter examines some of the problems people have encountered in cars, schools, offices, stores, and hotels.

AUTOMOBILES

Like a house, a car has a combustion system that is capable of producing carbon monoxide, a fuel storage and supply system that can leak, and carpeted and plastic surfaces that can off-gas. If we close the windows and run the heating or air conditioning, a car can be as much of an air envelope as any indoor environment. Fragrance emitters and cigarette smoke only add to the brew.

Cars, like houses, can get moldy. One fellow who was deeply in love with his rotary-engine sports car was despondent because he experienced allergy symptoms inside the vehicle when the heat was on. I took an air sample in the car with the heat off and then with the heat on. When the heat was on, the car was filled with mold spores. In this case the mold was growing in the damp carpet beneath the dashboard, and the spores were being dislodged and blown about by the airflow from the heater.

In other cars the spore source is moldy materials on or around the air conditioner's cooling coil. If the coil itself is covered with mold, the spores may not be released in the summer, when the coil is being used for air conditioning and is therefore damp. But in the winter, when the heating coil is used and the air conditioning coil is dry, look out! When the mold growth is dry, the spores more easily become airborne.

The heating and air conditioning systems of many vehicles have that tell-tale sweat sock odor from bacteria or yeast contamination or the earthy odor of mold. If your car has a suspicious odor, consider taking it to an air conditioning shop that will remove the entire system and clean it. Do not allow technicians to use caulks that have persistent odors, however, or you will have a new problem, as I once did in my car. If there are fibrous insulation materials near the coil, have them replaced if possible with nonfibrous insulation such as closed-cell foam. If automobile heating and cooling systems had filters that were 40 percent efficient, they would reduce the number of nutrients and therefore the level of biological growth. Unfortunately, as far as I know not many automobile manufacturers now have systems with filtration.

One woman called me from Virginia with an odd mold story. Her car had been rear-ended at a red light and had been repaired at a collision shop. Soon afterward the car developed a strong smell of mold. She was worried because her teenage daughter, who was allergic to mold, spent several hours each day in the car, commuting to school and to her other commitments. The girl was a straight-A student and a promising young athlete, but after the car was fixed she began to feel lethargic and developed dark rings around her eyes. Soon she was sleeping for long periods during the day and could not function effectively in school. When the mother persuaded her daughter to stop using the car, the girl immediately began to feel better. Within a few days her energy returned.

The mother inspected the car and found that the carpeting under the backseat was damp and the trunk contained several inches of water. I never saw the car, but most likely the damage was not properly repaired and rainwater was dripping into the trunk around the edges. I recommended that the family make the trunk leak-tight, replace all the carpeting in the car, clean the upholstery, and have the heating and air conditioning system professionally disinfected. (The system no doubt was contaminated, since it had been operating while all the mold was growing inside.) I believe the woman got rid of the mold and then sold the car anyway. Because a used car may have been in a flood or suffered other water damage, there are pitfalls in buying such a vehicle, particularly one with unexplained odors.

In another car, a station wagon with an odor of bacteria, water was leaking through the tailgate handle, dripping down within the door to the latch at the bottom, and soaking into the pad beneath the carpet in the storage area behind the backseat. Moisture was never visible because it entered surreptitiously from beneath the carpet pad.

One young man who called me was sickened by an irritating odor that seemed to emanate from his car trunk. The car was brand new, but the smell of burning rubber inside the vehicle made him feel so ill that he was considering trading the automobile in. He could not find the origin of the odor. Ultimately he and I discovered that the spare tire was the culprit. Sulfur (and sulfur compounds, which have strong odors) is used to harden the rubber in tires, and though the odor from most rubber products diminishes over time, some continue to off-gas the smell. We wrapped the entire rubber portion of the spare in heavy aluminum foil, and the odor diminished significantly.

Many malodorous compounds, including butenyl mercaptan (another sulfur compound that is responsible in part for skunk odor), are destroyed by ozone. There is a great deal of controversy about the use of ozone in occupied spaces. Just because ozone is a natural product of lightning doesn't mean it is safe. In fact, most authorities agree that ozone generators can be hazardous to one's health, and I would never recommend using ozone to deodorize a home while people are living there. The young man and I did, however, run an ozone generator in the unoccupied car for fifteen minutes to minimize the residual odor, now that the source was gone. The owner was quite pleased when he drove off (after airing out the interior for several minutes before he got in). Many people think that wrapping something smelly in plastic will contain the odor, but this often doesn't work. Most plastic bags are made of polyethylene, and so are the plastic lids on coffee cans. You can smell coffee right through the lid once the can is opened, because aroma molecules literally dissolve in the polyethylene at the inside of the cover, diffuse through, and evaporate at the top side (even after the cover is off the can, it will continue to off-gas coffee aroma for a short period). If you have an item you suspect is off-gassing, don't bother wrapping it in a polyethylene garbage bag to stop the odor. Use aluminum foil instead, and cover the item completely. Vapor molecules can't diffuse through foil because the metal is too dense and the spaces between the atoms are too small to allow the "larger" vapor molecules to penetrate.

In another car odor story, a couple took great pains to tell me how the smell in their automobile seemed to vary according to weather conditions, whether the windows were open or closed, the speed of the car, the wind, and so forth. At first I thought it peculiar that they described the situation to me in such detail, but then they told me they had been gathering data and trying to figure out the source for weeks. The couple lived nearby, and they drove the car over to my driveway so I could try to help them.

I asked the husband to sit in the car. Then I depressurized the interior by tightly shutting three of the four windows, inserting a vacuum cleaner hose in the fourth window, rolling that window up to the hose, and covering the gap with duct tape. As the vacuum cleaner pulled the air out of the car and lowered the pressure, only fresh air from the outside was forced in through the normal leakage pathways. As I "vacuumed," the husband sniffed around the interior of the car and recognized the offending smell as coming from the defroster vent. The most likely source was a rubber gasket inside the heating unit.

A former student of mine also had a car air quality problem. His own car was a "wreck," so when he had to make a long trip he would exchange vehicles with his father, who owned a newer car. On one occasion the father became so nauseated while he was driving his son's car that he had to abandon it and take a bus home. After that the son realized that he too often felt sick while driving the car.

Every time he ran the defroster, a film appeared on the window, and both father and son wondered if this might be contributing. Using a bright flashlight, I found that when the defroster was running, a mist of liquid was ejected from the defroster vents. The droplets consisted of radiator water containing permanent antifreeze (ethylene glycol). Beneath the glove compartment, we also noticed liquid dripping onto the carpet from the heater. Apparently the heater core (the heat exchanger in the car's heating system) was leaking, and the blower blades were spinning in a puddle of radiator fluid. The agitation created an aerosol of droplets that was then carried out the vents by the air-flow. The father had the heater core replaced and the car cleaned, and the problem was solved.

When I first started in the home inspection business, I drove a blue pickup that I had bought used. The truck was my office away from home and my home away from home. I booked appointments from the cellular phone and napped on the front seat whenever I had the chance between inspections. I often noticed a slight odor of gasoline in the cab, and when I drove I always felt better when the windows were open.

I used to use glass draw tubes to measure the carbon monoxide in buildings, and after one job I accidentally left an unused testing tube on the front seat. Something must have broken the end off and activated the tube. When I got out of the truck I found the tube on the seat, and it had changed color completely, indicating the presence of carbon monoxide. I then found that the exhaust system had been leaking gases and that the vapor capture system for gasoline fumes in the engine was broken. For months, both carbon monoxide and gasoline fumes had been filling the cab. It's unfortunate there are no carbon monoxide alarms for cars.

SCHOOLS

While I owned the blue pickup, I began to be very sensitive to chemicals and fragrances. I suspect my exposure to the carbon monoxide and gasoline fumes increased my susceptibility. I was originally educated as a chemist. In graduate school I was a teaching assistant in dozens of organic chemistry labs while groups of students (sometimes as many as sixty) boiled gallons of solvents. Vapors rose freely into the air. When ether was the solvent, we would leave the lab feeling tipsy. I was used to working with chemicals, and though I knew they could be toxic, I just didn't worry much about my exposure. Now I feel very differently.

College labs are also operated very differently now than when I was in graduate school. Solvents have to be handled in fume hoods that draw the chemical vapors upward and out of the building to the roof, where they are discharged. (Unfortunately there have been instances when hood exhausts were positioned too close to the fresh-air intakes on the roof and solvents were drawn back into the building!)

The irony is that although there are now stricter regulations about operating labs, there are not many building regulations regarding the use of cleaning fluids and paints that contain some of these same solvents. The environment in a space that is being painted or cleaned is sometimes not all that different from the environment in the lab when I was a teaching assistant. Even storing paint and cleaning compounds can cause problems if there is any leakage (see chapter 14).

If a school has a carpentry, automobile, welding, or printing shop or even an art studio or photography darkroom, sawdust and fumes can circulate in the air. In one high school the library was directly above the art studio, where students worked with oil paints and soaked their brushes in paint thinner. It took a year or two of exposure, but eventually the solvent fumes and odors from the drying oils began to make the librarian sick. Fumes from inadequately vented office machines such as copiers can also be troublesome (see chapter 13).

When we are on the subject of schools—or any indoor space where people congregate for long periods—we have to consider that people themselves emit many chemicals, some of them pollutants. Cigarette smokers emit a telltale odor from their skins and exhale it. And it's hard to hide the fact that you've had a glass of wine, because alcohol in the blood evaporates into the air in the lungs and is exhaled. This is the basis of the Breathalyzer test given to people suspected of driving under the influence.

You don't have to introduce substances into your body for them to be present in your breath, however. In metabolizing nutrients our bodies produce a number of chemicals, including acetone and butyric acid. We also exhale carbon dioxide and moisture that has evaporated from the lungs, raising the humidity in the spaces where we breathe. Bacteria in the moist and sweaty areas of our bodies add their own overtones. Air with elevated levels of human emission products (bioeffluents) makes a room seem stuffy and uncomfortable; we all notice this when we enter a poorly ventilated, crowded space. Some air quality researchers believe excessive bioeffluents are responsible for some sick building symptoms. Ventilation guidelines in larger buildings provide for 15 cubic feet (420 liters) of air per person per minute (15 cfm), in part to dilute these bioeffluents.

I was asked to look at one school building because parents had noticed changes in their children's health and behavior. One father told me his daughter used to come home and play every day after school, but now all she did was sleep. He also complained that all the children had been having more colds during the winter. When I visited the school I found that, to save energy, all the windows and fresh-air vents had been sealed with plastic sheets. There was so little air exchange that the moisture from the rooms' inhabitants was condensing on the plastic. It was a rainy day outside and in. The elevated moisture in the building was also exacerbating a very significant growth of mold. The newer portion of the school had been built slab on grade and was fully carpeted. On the day of my visit, children were running in dripping wet from the rain, dropping mud from their shoes onto the carpet. My Burkard air samples were full of mold hyphae.

The background level of carbon dioxide in fresh outside air is about 350 parts per million (ppm), and the recommended maximum level of carbon dioxide indoors is about 800 ppm. The levels I measured in certain classrooms were over 2,000 ppm, and some were over 3,000. These increased levels of carbon dioxide are not toxic, but people tend to feel sleepy when exposed to them.

Because there was less outside infiltration air to heat, the school's heating bills may have been cut in half that winter, but the families probably bore the cost through increased medical expenses. Once the ventilation system was reinstated, conditions improved. I also recommended removing the carpeting from the concrete and installing resilient tile, but I don't know whether these steps were taken.

Younger children have other risks of exposure in classrooms. It's not unusual, for example, to find rabbits or hamsters in kindergarten classrooms. I know it's hard to object, since children love furry pets, but if your child is allergic to these animals, don't let emotions win over common sense. Ask the school to remove the animals or assign your child to another classroom. If a child is experiencing allergy symptoms at school, the carpet dust should be tested for allergens.

One of my pet peeves is basement day care centers, which seem to be sprouting up everywhere like mushrooms: in church basements, community centers, the lower levels of office buildings, and even in homes. Like all basement spaces, these lower-level rooms are prone to mold and mite infestations, particularly if they are carpeted, as they most often are. (I discuss basement issues in detail in chapters 8 and 9.) If your son or daughter has allergies, it's not a good idea to have the child crawling alongside mites on a moldy carpet all day long.

Though air quality problems in school buildings are common, some occur intermittently. For example, when the bell rings to dismiss classes and students and teachers pour into the hallways, the dust levels increase dramatically. This is true in any building, but even more so if there are carpets. In day care centers, exposure to mold and other particulates from carpeting increases similarly during more active play. When carpets are not professionally washed, irritating detergents or other chemical residues may be left behind, and these too can become airborne with the particles they adhere to. There should not be wall-to-wall carpeting in school buildings, despite the acoustical advantages. I would rather have noise than mold, but I'm sure that in any given building, an acoustical engineer could make suggestions for noise abatement without the use of carpeting.

So what can you do about a potential air quality problem in a school building? For one thing, believe your child. If he or she is feeling ill or extraordinarily sleepy, there may be an IAQ problem. If anyone in your family has allergies, don't hesitate to object to the presence of animals in the room (remember, dander is carried on clothing). If the building is undergoing renovations, make sure the construction area is well contained. Ask about storage of cleaning compounds and about exhaust ventilation in shops, printing areas, offices, and so forth. Many classrooms have unit ventilators along the wall for heating or cooling. Check these with a flashlight and be sure you don't see layers of dust inside. And don't forget to find out whether other parents share your concerns.

Don't settle for a moldy carpeted basement classroom space. I know of one school that had its library in the basement. The space was welcoming, with brightly painted walls and comfortable, child-sized chairs here and there for quiet reading, but the librarian had to keep asking the children to stop coughing. If you suspect the carpet in your child's classroom is moldy, try the aluminum foil test (explained in chapter 6) for odor or have a laboratory test the dust for mold and mites.

Children and teachers spend hours every day in school buildings, so it's just as important to be vigilant about air quality there as in your own home. I recommend the EPA's action kit, "Indoor Air Quality: Tools for Schools" (see the resource guide at the end of the book), which offers parents and educators a practical plan for solving IAQ problems in school buildings.

THE WORKPLACE
Small Buildings

Many adults work in office buildings, and many of the same problems can occur there as in home offices (see chapter 13). Unusual situations can occur, however. One woman, a psychologist, had been seeing clients in a basement office for fifteen years, and in the past three years she had been experiencing increasing health reactions. Within a few hours of entering her office, she would grow hoarse and develop a headache. She fought off three bouts of pneumonia in one year, saw many physicians, and had a lung biopsy. I found a very strong odor of tar in her office, and I lifted the carpet to see if there was an odor source within the floor. Indeed, under the ancient linoleum was black roofing paper. We removed a sample of this paper and took it outside, where she sniffed it and immediately identified it as the source of the odor. There was another problem: I found with a Burkard sampler that there was *Penicillium* mold growth in the carpet, probably because the floor was over a dirt crawl space.

I don't know whether she was having a toxic reaction to the phenolic emissions from the tar paper or was responding to the allergens or toxins from the mold spores. In any case, when she had the old flooring removed and new carpeting installed, her symptoms disappeared.

Large Buildings

I was asked to look at a computer room in a large office building because some employees suffered allergy symptoms there. It was a scene from a science fiction movie. The floor was a raised metal grid, and I could see into the space below, where the cables connecting the machines to one another were strung.

The windowless room had only one door and contained its own air conditioning system, along with a large humidifier to keep the relative humidity high enough to prevent electrostatic charges from building up. The humidifier had an air intake at the top, covered with a media filter two inches thick, a water reservoir inside for evaporating moisture into the air, and a blower at the bottom that discharged the humidified air into the space below.

The room was so packed with walls of flashing lights and boards that it felt like an electronics canyon. Because this room was the processing center for a large business, I was very nervous about moving or even touching anything. I could feel air movement everywhere because of the continuous circulation from the blowers. I took my usual three-minute Burkard sample of the air and was surprised to find it was the cleanest I had ever seen, probably because very few people spent time in the room and the air was constantly being filtered. With a microscope, I could see that the only particles present appeared to be respirable (less than 0.0001 inch or 2.5 micron) rust crystals, though I could not be certain just by looking. A sample I took with sticky tape of the dust from the top of the humidifier filter contained many similar particles.

To identify the particles, I took the tape sample to a scanning electron microscope laboratory, where I found that most consisted of rust. The source of the rust was the interior of the humidifier itself, where water was causing components to corrode. The first thing I noted when I entered the computer room was a slight wet sponge odor. I can only assume that bacteria were growing in the water reservoir and that products of this biological growth were adhering to the rust, which was then being aerosolized in the strong airflows. If the walls of the water reservoirs had been plastic, they would not have corroded. I recommended that the reservoir be disinfected periodically and that the humidifier filter be made airtight at the edges and be changed more often. As long as no nutrients entered the water, biological growth would be minimized.

What are the other sources of contamination in large office buildings? There are many, including new furniture and office partitions, which, as discussed in chapters 2 and 13, can off-gas formaldehyde. Office copiers and printers can also be sources of irritating chemicals (see chapter 13). The plastic in new computer monitors and communications cables can emit irritants. One common source of eye, skin, and lung irritation is self-copy paper, also called carbonless copy paper, commonly used with memos, bills, and other forms. Some people who touch the forms have allergic reactions, and others who are highly sensitized may experience asthma symptoms in a room where the forms are being processed in large numbers because particulates with chemicals are aerosolized.

Wall-to-wall carpeting, so common in large buildings, is another source of contamination. Properly vacuumed, washed, and maintained carpeting can be of minimal concern, but all too often carpeting is not well maintained or becomes damp from leaks, weather intrusion, food spills, and improper washing. I investigated one office building in which several people who worked in one corner of one floor were having asthma symptoms. Because of improperly installed flashing, a significant amount of water was coming through the exterior walls. The carpeting and drywall had soaked up the water, mold was proliferating, and *Stachybotrys* was growing on the drywall. Deteriorating wool fibers and chemical off-gassing are also concerns (see chapters 1, 5, and 9 for detailed discussions of carpeting). Some of the particulate emissions from carpeting can be minimized by using HEPA-filtered vacuums. If carpet dust bothers you, try to have the building's maintenance staff use only HEPA vacuums.

Although I dislike wall-to-wall carpeting, I believe the largest cause of sick building symptoms is contaminated air handling equipment. Every teaspoon of air we inhale in a large building has been circulated through heating and cooling coils and, in some cases, through hundreds of feet of ductwork. Even if only a short portion of the air conveyance pathway is covered with biological growth, allergens and other irritants can become airborne. I have sampled hundreds of air conditioning coils and their neighboring fiberglass liners, and I have never found any that lacked some form of biological growth (mold, bacteria, or yeast), because air conditioning lowers the temperature of air and thus increases relative humidity.

Unfortunately this condition is so widespread that it is considered acceptable by most people who maintain the mechanical equipment in buildings. Some systems are so contaminated with years of accumulated "bioslime" that the sludge has to be shoveled out. For people who are highly sensitized, however, almost no level of bioslime is acceptable.

If you work in a large building that has a sweat sock or mold odor associated with the mechanical system, you must insist the source be eliminated.

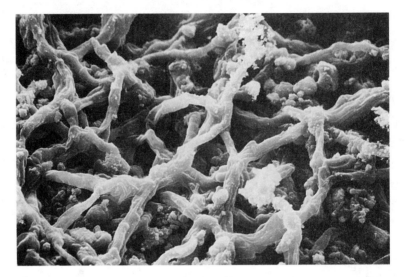

FIGURE 16.1. Mold hyphae on an air conditioning coil. The chief executive of a computer company was experiencing allergy symptoms in his office. A sample of dust taken from the front of his air conditioning coil was infiltrated by a vast network of mold hyphae. (1,500× SEM)

This will usually entail costly, scrupulous cleaning and disinfecting of the heat exchange coils and drip trays and possibly replacing fiberglass lining materials that contain biological growth. Although using them is common practice, in my opinion fibrous lining materials should not be anywhere near cooling coils. All mechanical equipment in buildings should be readily accessible and its location identified. The dates of filter changes should be color-coded so that anyone can tell just by looking how old a filter is. Only media or equivalently efficient filters should be used, and filters should be installed whenever possible to prevent any unfiltered air from reaching the coils. (Even if only a small portion of the air leaks around a filter, significant amounts of dust can accumulate on the coil.) As I noted in chapter 10, typical fiberglass filters used on smaller units by most maintenance companies are virtually useless.

An office in another building I investigated had, on a single floor, twenty heat pumps hung above suspended ceiling tiles. Each heat pump was supposed to have its own fiberglass filter, but some were missing. Each pump also had its own contaminated heat exchange coil. Because the maintenance work was of considerable magnitude, the threat to indoor air quality was a concern.

Another drawback with this arrangement of suspended heat pumps (common in newer buildings) is the lack of ducted returns. In nearly all cases the ceiling plenum serves as the shared return. Thus contaminants from the space between the floor and ceiling, or irritants contained in any one of the heat pumps, can be circulated throughout the office.

Ultimately, I think we should be dehumidifying our buildings in addition to cooling them with air conditioning. In a typical building, the cooling system's trigger for turning on and off is determined by the temperature set on the thermostat rather than by the relative humidity of the air. Thus the air conditioning, which does remove moisture, might nonetheless shut down when the temperature is 70°F and the relative humidity is 70 percent—uncomfortable conditions and very conducive to mold growth. If the relative humidity was controlled by a dehumidistat, then the system would continue to operate until the humidity was lowered to the setting. Maintaining buildings below 60 percent (preferably closer to 50 percent) relative humidity during the cooling season would minimize mildew.

Adequate ventilation is another vital concern in a big building. Ventilation systems are supposed to supply fresh air to every floor while removing an equal proportion of stale air and exhausting it out of the building. In fact, if there were no air exchange (fresh air in, stale air out), breathing inside that building would be no different from breathing into a plastic bag. With enough occupants, the carbon dioxide concentration would rise and the oxygen concentration would drop until breathing at all would become difficult. Eventually, in a truly closed system, the lack of oxygen would be lethal; fortunately, no building is this airtight.

Even in ventilated buildings, areas of the building may appear to have stale air, perhaps owing to poor distribution of the fresh air, which is often introduced at only one location. Other IAQ problems have occurred because the fresh-air intakes were above the loading docks, where diesel trucks idled, or on the roof near plumbing vent stacks, so that sewer gas was entrained. Even worse, some fresh-air intakes are downwind from cooling towers that contain warm water and therefore are possibly contaminated with *Legionella* bacteria, the cause of Legionnaires' disease. I heard of one fresh-air intake that was in an underground parking garage, so carbon monoxide and car exhaust were entrained.

Current ASHRAE (American Society of Heating, Refrigerating, and Air-Conditioning Engineers) guidelines recommend that about 15 cubic feet (420 liters) of air per minute be supplied for each occupant of a building, but this recommended quantity of ventilation air for buildings has varied over time. At one time it was about 5 cubic feet (140 liters) of air per minute per person. Over the past decade, many researchers have looked into IAQ problems (sick building syndrome) in larger buildings and have pointed to inadequate ventilation as the cause.

One study set out to determine if changing the ventilation rate in buildings would make a noticeable difference in employee symptoms and IAQ complaints. The researchers designed a very complete questionnaire, which was administered several times to every person in the buildings under study as the ventilation rates were increased and decreased. None of the workers were aware that the ventilation rates were doubled between one week and the next. The study found there was no significant difference in the level of complaints and concluded that ventilation was far less important than people had assumed.

These results were widely reported in the news because they seemed to contradict the common perception about the cause of sick building syndrome. Few people realized, however, what the study really showed. All the buildings that were included in the research had initial ventilation rates of at least 20 cubic feet (560 liters) of air per minute per person, more than the current recommended guideline. The ventilation was never reduced to rates I would consider inadequate, so the sensible conclusion is that 20 cubic feet of air per minute is more than enough for comfort.

One reason for increasing ventilation is to dilute volatile organic compounds found in emissions from furnishings, carpeting, plastics, or office machines. It's particularly important that when renovations are undertaken the areas be isolated and have increased ventilation. Air that is exhausted from a space under construction should not be mixed with air for the rest of the building. I know many individuals who have become sensitized or ill from prolonged exposure to elevated concentrations of solvents in buildings during renovation and construction, or during other repeated activities such as cleaning, painting, or pesticide application. Ventilation rates have to be adjusted according to the building's occupancy and use.

Sick building syndrome has also been referred to as tight building syndrome, with the assumption that the building is sick because there is inadequate fresh air. This may be the case in buildings where concentrations of volatile organic compounds are elevated. In most sick buildings, though, *I believe that bioaerosols are most often responsible for some of the building occupants' symptoms and that increasing the ventilation rates will not necessarily solve the problem.* Blaming an air quality problem on the building's energy-saving design is a way both to accept the conditions as inevitable and to avoid questioning maintenance practices.

If you are suffering from IAQ problems in a building where you work, I recommend you acquire the EPA's "Building Air Quality: A Guide for Building Owners and Facility Managers" (see the resource guide). This publication contains practical guidance for maintenance in large buildings, information for diagnosing and solving indoor air quality problems, and a list of such agencies as the Occupational Safety and Health Administration (OSHA) and the National Institute for Occupational Safety and Health (NIOSH). If the management or the owner is not responding to your concerns, you may want to request a transfer to another space or building. As a last resort, you may have to find a new job.

ALLERGENS ADHERING TO AIRBORNE PARTICLES

I believe that in many sick buildings, nonbioaerosol particulates such as soot and plaster dust have been coated with allergens from biological growth. In fact one Norwegian study demonstrated that particles of airborne soot in homes where there are cats are coated with cat allergens. This can make it hard to discover the sources of IAQ problems. I can see a soot particle under a microscope, and I can see cat dander under a microscope, but I have no way of seeing cat allergens on soot or mold allergens or mycotoxins on plaster particles, because mycotoxin molecules, and the proteins that make up most allergens, are too small to be seen with a microscope.

For example, in one building I theorized that allergens from mold may have been transferred to the surface of paint pigment particles. I found extraordinarily high levels of submicron paint pigment particles in the air samples I took in the building. I don't know where these particles originated; perhaps the interior had been spray painted. It seemed to me that the particles had

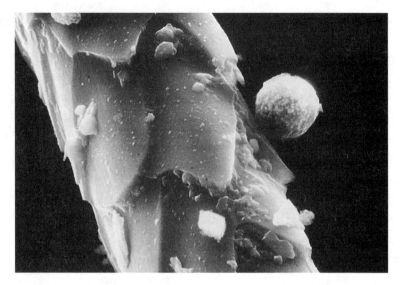

FIGURE 16.2. Spray paint on a cat hair. A microscopic sphere of spray paint sits on the surface of a cat hair. Such spheres may contain hundreds of paint pigment particles and commonly occur in a large range of sizes in buildings that have been spray painted. Under certain conditions, the sphere may break up and release the pigment particles onto a surface or into a liquid containing allergens. If the particles then become airborne, they may become infinitely small carriers of allergens. (2,000× SEM)

been recirculated throughout the rooms many times. I also found mold spores (which are many times larger) that were covered with paint pigment particles. The level of mold spores was not extraordinarily high, and in themselves the pigment particles would not have been of concern except that an occupant's asthma symptoms were increasing. If they had been in or on a contaminated surface, such as the ten-year-old furnace filter that was covered with pigment particles and growing mold, some of the numerous particles may have become carriers of allergens.

Latex allergy, one example of known allergen transfer, can be life-threatening, particularly among nurses—about 10 percent are affected. It is believed that latex allergy is acquired by contact with latex hospital gloves and is exacerbated by inhaling starch granules from the gloves. These gloves are made from an emulsion—the milky liquid secretion of rubber trees (*Hevea brasiliensis*)—that contains oily microscopic droplets of latex in water. Dissolved in the emulsion are molecules of proteins that are far smaller than the oily droplets.

When the latex is processed into gloves, some of the proteins remain on the surface, even though the gloves are washed before packaging for sale. Clean latex rubber tends to stick to itself; to prevent the gloves from doing this, they are dusted with cornstarch "donning" powder, which consists of starch granules of about 0.0004 to 0.001 inch (10 to 25 microns). Because the granules are small and are in physical contact with the gloves' surface, they acquire some of the latex proteins, several of which have been identified as allergens. When people put on the gloves, clouds of cornstarch granules become airborne and are readily inhaled.

With a microscope, I can't see a difference between a cornstarch granule that has latex allergens on it and one that doesn't, because the protein molecules are too small. Fortunately, however, dust can be chemically tested for latex allergens. Unfortunately, most of the thousands of other allergens that might be adhering to any of the millions of airborne particulates can be detected only by the reactions of the building's inhabitants.

VACATIONS

Time and time again people have told me that hotel and motel rooms have made them feel sick, and not because of the price (though sometimes that can seem reason enough!). In hot, humid parts of the country, the rooms are so prone to mold growth that the places could be called Mildew Motels. Even in colder climates, contaminated air conditioning units are the rule rather than the exception. In some motels, rooms are around a central indoor pool. This may be relaxing for some, but those who react to chlorine should avoid rooms like this, particularly if the windows to the exterior don't open.

Hotels and motels are often redecorated while they are still open for guests, and paint fumes and other chemicals mix with the indoor air. A dear friend walked by a room in which new carpeting was being glued down. Her larynx swelled in response to the vapors from the adhesive that were drifting out into the hallway, and she lost her voice. She couldn't even complain to the manager! No matter what the cosmetic state of your rented room, the bedding can cause problems if it is contaminated with mites and mold or if it contains down and you are sensitized.

Be a critical shopper and view the hotel room before moving in. Ask for a nonsmoking room, but don't assume it until you check. Don't use air conditioning or heaters with blowers unless you must, and carry an N95 NIOSH fine-particle mask with you just in case. Be cautious about having housekeeping vacuum the room, because this may kick up irritating dust; and don't let them spray fragrances around your room. In fact, if you don't mind making your own bed and straightening up the bathroom, keep housekeeping out altogether. If you have allergies or asthma, traveling with your own pillow isn't a bad idea.

To go on vacation, you have to travel. We've discussed cars already, but planes and trains can also have air conditioning and heating systems, as well as carpets and furnishings, that are contaminated. You may also find yourself close to someone who wears a heavy fragrance or carries dander or mite allergens. If you are bothered, move to another seat or wear your particle mask. You may look a little strange, but it's better than having an asthma attack during your vacation.

Although you don't have the same control over the conditions in office buildings, schools, hotels, and retail shops as you have in your own home, it's important to have a clear idea of some of the IAQ issues in these other environments. You can then better protect yourself and be a more effective advocate for healthier air.

RECOMMENDATIONS

AUTOMOBILE

- Don't smoke or use fragrance emitters in your car.
- If there is a strong odor from your car's air conditioning system, have the system professionally cleaned. Replace fiberglass insulation with closed-cell foam insulation.
- If there is moldy carpeting in your car, replace the carpet and the pad.

- If you see a liquid film from your defroster, have the heater core checked for leaks.
- Maintain your car's exhaust system and fuel line.

SCHOOLS

- If your child is allergic to an animal, be sure one is not kept as a pet in the classroom.
- Get a copy of the EPA's action kit "Indoor Air Quality: Tools for Schools" (see the resource guide).
- Be sure that the interiors of unit ventilators (a type of heating unit with a blower, usually installed along the wall), are free of dust, that the filters are installed properly, and that the fresh-air vents are operating.
- Promote classrooms free of wall-to-wall carpeting.

THE WORKPLACE

- Purchase a copy of the EPA's "Building Air Quality: A Guide for Building Owners and Facility Managers" (see the resource guide).
- If there are odors, try to identify the sources as a first step to eradication.
- Machines that emit chemicals should have adequate exhaust ventilation.
- Be sure HEPA vacuums are used for carpet cleaning.
- All air handling equipment (e.g., blowers, air conditioning coils, condensate pans) should be kept clean (free of all dust) and well maintained.
- If possible, be sure the best possible (media) filters are used in HVAC systems and that they are changed as needed.
- In damp climates, attempt to control humidity rather than just temperature.
- Relative humidity should be maintained below 60 percent, preferably close to 50 percent.

- Fresh-air intakes should not be in areas where contaminants can be entrained.
- If you enter a building where bioaerosols bother you, either leave or wear an N95 NIOSH fine-particle mask.

TRAVEL

- Before committing to a hotel or motel, check the room. If it bothers you, try another room or leave.
- Try to stay in motels or hotels where the room windows can be opened to the exterior.
- Travel with your own pillow and an N95 NIOSH fine-particle mask.
- Don't operate a moldy room air conditioning or heating unit.
- If you have allergies to dust or fragrances, don't let housekeeping vacuum or use sprays in the room during your stay.

Closing Remarks: Take Charge

Up to now, we've looked at a litany of house problems: one disaster after another, occurring in various rooms of a home. Woven throughout have been stories of people's suffering. I'll admit it's been a pretty grim collection.

A friend who has severe allergies offered to read the rough draft of this book and provide some comments. I was particularly interested in her reactions, because in my mind she is just the sort of person I'm hoping to reach. She told me she tried to read herself to sleep with the first few chapters. What a mistake! The more she read, the wider awake she was. When she imagined dust mites nibbling on skin scales under her sheets, she had to put the manuscript down or risk insomnia.

If you read this book and then go out and purchase a HEPA vacuum, I'll be pleased; but if you throw out your couch or your mattress, I'll be upset. I wrote the book not to cause hysteria, but to help people suffering from allergies and asthma gain greater control over the air quality where they live, play, and work. I believe firmly that taking simple steps can make enormous improvements, just as minor omissions can create major problems.

Your home won't contain all the trouble spots identified in this book. Your story won't be the same as the stories of people I've discussed here. But if you are having asthma or allergy symptoms in your home, then I hope some of the information I've given will help you begin to exercise greater control by identifying and eradicating some of the sources of indoor air quality problems. The following steps should guide you in your crusade.

BELIEVE YOUR BODY

If you have headaches or rashes, if you sneeze or cough, or if you have trouble breathing when you are in certain spaces, believe what your body is telling you. Even if someone standing next to you has none of the symptoms you are experiencing and thinks you may be imagining things, trust your own nose and believe your own lungs. The first step toward taking charge is accepting that we are all different and that we respond to our environments in individual ways.

STUDY YOUR BODY'S REACTIONS

Be a scientist and objectively observe how your body responds to its environment. Is there any relation between the symptoms you experience and the place you are in or the activity around you? Do you have particular difficulty at certain times of the day, in certain seasons of the year (when the heat or air conditioning is on, for example), or under certain weather conditions (rain, wind)? Do you cough more frequently when one of your friends is near you? Keep a journal so you can notice patterns. Don't be discouraged if it's hard to make connections between what you're feeling and what may be happening around you—some people have allergic reactions only hours after coming in contact with irritants. Use your journal to identify any relation between your symptoms and the environmental conditions where you live and work.

IDENTIFY AND REMOVE PROBABLE SOURCES OF IRRITANTS

Once you have identified specific areas of your home that may be causing problems, use this book as a room-by-room guide to remove some of the sources of irritants.

TURN TO A PROFESSIONAL WHEN NECESSARY

Sometimes the causes of IAQ problems are so complicated and interconnected that a professional is needed to help you make sense of the evidence. It's always better to turn to an expert than to be misled into doubting your body's reactions. Be careful, though, to depend on someone who knows what he or she is doing. One man with asthma called me after he had employed two "environmental testing companies" to determine whether his home had air quality problems. These companies tested for benzene, ammonia, formaldehyde, and carbon monoxide and measured relative humidity and temperature, but they never looked for any allergens or irritants that might have caused asthma. I found mold and mites in the carpet in the finished basement.

Over the many years I've been in this business, I've received numerous messages from people who have followed the advice I'm offering here. Words like *relief* and *improvement* occur again and again. "Things are much better now," wrote one client; another wrote, "I gained confidence by solving the problem in the right way." One man reported by e-mail: "Your suggestions made a lot of difference. We replaced the carpets with hardwood and the hot-air heating system with forced hot water, removed or sealed all the old ducts and vents, discontinued the use of the wood stove, and completely cleaned the basement." This man did a lot of work, but sometimes just removing a moldy rug, getting rid of smelly window screens, replacing the down quilt with a synthetic-filled puff, or cleaning a heating or cooling system can make an enormous difference.

Let me share one client's promising story. She was a perfectly healthy middle-aged social worker who had purchased a condominium in a new building. She had led an active life, but after living in her new home for several years, she found it increasingly hard to find the energy to exercise. She also began to have difficulty concentrating at work. By the end of her seventh year in the condo, she had taken a leave of absence from her job and was barely able to lift herself from her couch. She had also acquired a chronic cough and asthma.

I found many sources of contaminants in her home, and a doctor confirmed that she had severe allergies to mold. She cleaned up her home environment, and most of her symptoms disappeared. Yet when she tried to return to work she became ill again and was forced to remain on leave. She insisted there was mold in the basement office she occupied, which her employer denied until the soggy, moldy ceiling tiles above her desk collapsed under their own weight. Now that her condo is cleaned up and she remains away from the office, the woman's health has vastly improved. She has also become a more active advocate for her own well-being. For example, she now has a sharper sense of when her symptoms reappear. If she walks into a store or other indoor space and feels bad, she leaves. And I don't think she will agree to work in a basement office again.

Her battle to keep her health continues daily, and periodically she updates me on her progress. She has many good days, but sometimes when contractors are working in her building and generating dust, even on other floors, she finds conditions intolerable. Her office, which she can no longer enter, continues to have air quality problems. On one occasion former coworkers told her they got sick after moldy files from cabinets in her basement office were spread out on the first floor to "air" out.

I hesitated to use this story as the last one in the book, because it doesn't have a very happy ending. I was tempted to substitute a tale where a client proclaimed complete liberation from symptoms, but such a final account seems unrealistic. If you are sensitized to contaminants in your home, cleaning them up should make a big difference in your life. There is no way to guarantee that everything you are sensitized to will be eliminated from your indoor environment, however, or that you will not encounter allergens again during work or travel. My client is living a much better life because of the changes she was able to make in her home. Unfortunately, an entire world around her condominium is filled with unsympathetic listeners, poorly qualified technicians, and conditions beyond her control.

Even in my own home the struggle is ongoing. In the past month I have had to abandon office chairs with mite infestations and rugs that emitted wool dander. After some visitors leave, the only way for me to stop coughing is to open several doors and windows to air out the house. At least I know I'm not crazy, because I have seen the irritants that haunt me on a glass slide. For many of you this will not be true. The irritants and allergens may appear to be phantoms, but they are real, and you must believe you can eliminate many of them if you try.

This book may not provide a miracle cure, but I hope it will help you gain a better understanding of yourself and make you more confident that you can control your environment. If I've helped you, you might help others in turn by sharing your own success story. Don't be like that woman who said on my voice mail, "My house is killing me." Trust yourself. Make the effort and begin to take charge.

GLOSSARY

Acaricide: A chemical (usually benzyl benzoate or a borate) used to control mites.

Actinomycete: An organism that produces small spores and grows like mold but is actually a filamentous bacterium.

Adsorb: To collect onto a solid surface, usually from a vapor state. Adsorbed water is invisible and is always present as long as there is water vapor in the air.

Aerosol: Any suspended airborne particulate.

Aflatoxins: A series of toxic chemicals (mycotoxins) produced by molds. Produced by *Aspergillus flavus,* aflatoxin B_1 is a potent carcinogen and may be responsible for liver cancer in regions where contaminated grains are abundant.

Allergen: Anything that causes an allergic reaction. Many allergens are proteins. Cat and dog dander, mold spores, pollen, and dust mite fecal pellets all contain protein allergens.

Allergenco air sampler: A device that separates particulates such as pollen and mold spores from the air in which they are suspended. The particulates are trapped on a greased microscope slide. Sample times and intervals can be programmed, and multiple samples can be taken on the same slide.

Alternaria: A genus of fungi with large spores that generally contain allergens. One allergenic species, *Alternaria alternata,* is frequently found in house dust.

Amine: A nitrogen-containing class of organic chemicals related to ammonia. Amines are added to boiler water to minimize rust accumulation. Many amines are irritating or have a "fishy" smell. Cadaverine and putrescine are two malodorous amines produced by bacterial decomposition of muscle and other protein.

Anaphylaxis: A life-threatening allergic response.

Andersen sampler: An air-sampling instrument that uses petri dishes for determining the concentration of "live" (viable) mold spores in the air.

Asbestos: A naturally occurring carcinogenic mineral that exists in several forms, including amosite, chrysotile, and crocidolite. Chrysotile, believed to be the least carcinogenic form of asbestos, was used in thousands of products including insulation and construction composites.

ASHI: American Society of Home Inspectors, a professional, nonprofit association that provides a code of ethics and standards of practice.

Aspergillus: A genus of allergenic fungi. The spores grow in chains that are usually attached to a globular structure. *Aspergillus* is frequently found in homes with damp basements. One species, *Aspergillus fumigatus,* is associated with a lung disease called aspergillosis.

Bacharach Monoxor II: An instrument containing an air pump that is used to measure the concentration of carbon monoxide in the air.

Bacteria: Usually single-celled microscopic organisms that reproduce by division. Some bacteria are round; others are rod shaped or spiral. Bacteria cause syphilis, pneumonia, tuberculosis, infections of the skin, and many other diseases.

Bioaerosol: Any suspended particulate in the air that comes from a living organism. Bioaerosol can consist of pollen, mold spores, human and animal dander, insect body parts, and fecal material.

Bioeffluents: The chemicals produced by natural processes on and in the human body that can pollute the air in an indoor space.

Booklouse: A small nonbiting insect in the biological family Psocidae (psocids) that subsists on house dust.

Borescope: An optical instrument consisting of a long tube and a light, used for seeing into cavities.

Budding: The process by which yeast reproduces asexually. A small part of the parent cell forms a "bud" that enlarges and then separates and forms a new individual cell.

Burkard air sampler: A device that separates particulates such as pollen and mold spores from the air in which they are suspended. The particulates are trapped on a greased microscope slide.

Butyric acid: An unpleasant-smelling acid with the odor of stomach contents, produced by digestion of fats. Butyric acid is found in rancid butter and in perspiration, where it is produced by bacteria. Ceiling tiles made from cellulose (paper) contaminated with butyric acid have caused sick building symptoms and building odor problems.

Carbon monoxide: A colorless, odorless combustion gas that in low concentrations causes headaches and nausea and in high concentrations can cause coma and death.

Chase: A vertical space created to house pipes or ducts. A chase can be open from the basement all the way up to the attic.

Chemical change: A change in matter that produces one or more new substances. Thermal decomposition, digestion, and chemical reactions between substances are all chemical changes. Grinding, melting, and boiling are physical, not chemical changes.

Chemical sensitivity: An increased sensitivity to chemicals and other irritants found in the environment. Symptoms may include respiratory distress, muscle pain, headache, fatigue, neurological problems, and cognitive difficulties.

Chloramine: A toxic chemical produced when ammonia and chlorine bleach are mixed.

Chlordane: A persistent chlorinated hydrocarbon pesticide, often noticeable because of its odor. Now banned, chlordane was once used as a treatment for termites.

Chlorinated hydrocarbon: Generally, a compound containing the elements carbon, hydrogen, and chlorine, typically used as a solvent or pesticide.

Chronic fatigue syndrome (CFS):   A syndrome characterized by extreme and constant fatigue, thought to be caused by an immune system disorder. CFS is possibly linked to environmental triggers, such as viral infections and mold. Symptoms include impairment of short-term memory, sore throat, and joint pains.

Cladosporium: The most common genus of outdoor fungi. Spores of some species are allergenic, and others contain a mycotoxin, epicladosporic acid. Two species, *Cladosporium cladosporioides* and *C. herbarum,* grow well at low temperatures and can be found living in the dusts in air conditioning systems.

Closed-cell foam: A foam in which each "bubble space" is separate from every other one. Gas cannot be squeezed out of closed-cell foams, and they don't absorb water the way open-cell foams do. In an open-cell foam such as a sponge, all the bubble spaces are connected. When the foam is compressed, the gas is forced out.

Combustion chamber liner: A refractory (high temperature melting) material, usually ceramic, placed in the combustion chamber of an oil-fired furnace or boiler. The liner shields the metal from the intense heat of the flame.

Composite: A mixture of two or more materials whose properties are different from those of the separate ingredients.

Compound: A chemical combination of elements in a fixed atomic ratio. For example, carbon dioxide is a compound of carbon and oxygen in a one-to-two atomic ratio, written CO_2. Carbon monoxide is a compound of carbon and oxygen in a one-to-one atomic ratio (CO).

Condensate pump: A small pump and reservoir containing a float switch. The pump is used with air conditioning equipment to collect and eliminate water condensed from the air during cooling. Condensate pumps may also be used to eliminate water from high efficiency gas furnaces and dehumidifiers.

Condensate tray: A shallow metal tray tipped to a drain opening beneath an air conditioning coil to collect condensed water.

Condensation: A change of state from gas (vapor) to liquid; the opposite of evaporation. Clouds and fog form from condensation of water vapor to liquid water droplets in air. In a bathroom after someone has showered, the haze on a mirror is formed by condensation of water vapor onto a surface.

Conditioned air: Air that has been heated or cooled to the comfort range.

Conduction: Energy transferred by collisions, usually between "atomic" particles (electrons, atoms, molecules). Conduction occurs in all three phases of matter and is the principal method of heat energy transfer through solids (for example, a metal pot on a stove transfers heat from the burner to the food inside the pot).

Containment: A means by which dust is contained during the mitigation of a contaminated area, usually involving (among other steps) isolation of the space with plastic sheeting, cleaning with HEPA vacuums, and depressurization of the space with HEPA-filtered exhausts.

Convection: Heat transfer associated with bulk movements of matter owing to differences in density. Convection takes place only in gases and liquids, not in solids.

Copper arsenate: A compound of copper, arsenic, and oxygen in pressure-treated wood that is toxic to plants and animals as well as to fungi and bacteria.

Creosote: An oily liquid with a powerful odor produced when wood is burned or heated and used with solvent to preserve telephone poles and railroad ties.

Damper: A movable obstruction built into a pipe or duct to vary the flow of air or gases.

Dehumidistat: A variable control that senses relative humidity and regulates the operation of a dehumidifier.

Density: The amount of mass per unit volume. Oil floats on water because the two don't mix and because oil is less dense than water.

Dermatophytes: Fungi that cause skin conditions such as dermatitis and dandruff. Species include *Pityrosporum ovale* and *P. orbiculare*.

Dew point: The temperature at which water vapor in the air condenses to liquid water on a surface that is cooler than the air.

Diffuser: A round metal louver, usually in the ceiling, that spreads out the flow of air from a duct in an air conditioning or hot-air heating system.

Downdrafting: Airflow down instead of up a chimney flue.

"Dry" steam: Pure water vapor at or above 212°F, containing no liquid water.

Dust mite.   *See* Mites.

Electronic filter: A highly efficient filter that works on the principle of attracting charged particles using opposite-charged electrodes. Electronic filters cease to function when dirty.

Emulsion: A stable mixture of two or more immiscible liquids. Cream, for example, is primarily an emulsion of microscopic butterfat droplets in water.

Entrain: To draw in ("to go aboard").

Enzymes: Chemicals, usually protein, synthesized by an organism to facilitate chemical reactions. Enzymes help organisms digest protein, carbohydrate, and fat. Some enzymes are used within cells, and others are secreted to be used outside the cells.

EPA: The U.S. Environmental Protection Agency, a division of the federal government concerned with air quality, among other issues.

Epicoccum: A genus of allergenic molds with large brown spores. Chronic inhalation of *Epicoccum* spores is associated with increased respiratory problems.

Epinephrine: A hormone produced by the adrenal glands and used in emergency treatment of severe allergic reactions (anaphylaxis) to insect bites or foods.

Ethylene glycol: A toxic, barely volatile, and sweet-tasting chemical used to lower the freezing point of water.

Evaporation: A change of state from liquid to gas; the opposite of condensation.

Exfiltration: Pressure-driven flow of air out of a building or other defined space; the opposite of infiltration.

Fan coil: A device that provides heated or cooled air. A fan coil consists of one or more heat exchange coils and a blower.

Fascia board: A vertical trim board parallel to the edge of a roof but perpendicular to the soffit board.

Fiberglass: A nonwoven mixture of threadlike fibers made from molten glass and often held together by microscopic droplets of glue.

Fin tube: A copper pipe with numerous parallel aluminum plates (fins) attached. In a forced hot-water heating system, hot water is pumped through the copper pipe. Heat from the water is transferred to the copper and from there to the fins. Air between the fins is heated and rises by convection.

Flame roll-out: A flame that appears on the outside of a combustion chamber when a gas appliance is lit. Many conditions can cause flame roll-out, including inadequate draft and delayed ignition of the gas.

Flashing: Metal or other material used in construction to make watertight a joint or intersection that is exposed to rain.

Formaldehyde: An extremely irritating gas, very soluble in water. Formaldehyde off-gasses from adhesives found in some wood composites such as fiberboard.

Fungus (pl. fungi): A plantlike life form that lacks chlorophyll and thus depends on other living or dead organisms for its nourishment. Fungi include mushrooms and microscopic molds.

Gas: One of the three states of matter (gas, liquid, and solid). Most (but not all) gases are colorless and can't be seen.

Genus: A category of biological classification comprising various species.

Glow plug: An electric heating element that ignites the burner in an oven without a pilot light.

Glucan (beta-glucan): A component of the cell wall of all molds. Respirable bits of mold cell walls cause inflammation in the lung when inhaled.

Gram, milligram, and microgram: Measures of mass. There are one thousand micrograms in a milligram and one thousand milligrams in a gram. A U.S. copper penny has a mass of about three grams.

Grille: An opening in the floor, ceiling, or wall at the end of a return duct in a hot-air heating system. Unlike a register, a grille does not usually have a damper and cannot be closed.

Guanine: A water-insoluble substance that is the major component in the excretions of some animals, including birds (*guano* means bird droppings) and insects.

Heat exchanger: A device that either adds or takes away heat from a fluid that flows through it. The radiator on a car is a heat exchanger that transfers excess engine heat to the outside air. An air conditioning coil is a heat exchanger that cools the circulated air by removing heat from it.

HEPA vacuum: A vacuum cleaner with a high efficiency particulate arrestance (HEPA) filter. A HEPA filter is supposed to remove 99.97 percent of 0.3 micron particulates from the air flowing through it and 100 percent of the particulates larger than 1 micron.

Histoplasmosis: A lung disease caused by a fungus, *Histoplasma capsulatum*, found in bird droppings.

Humidistat: A variable control that senses relative humidity and regulates the operation of a humidifier.

HVAC: Heating, ventilating, and air conditioning.

Hydrocarbon: A compound of carbon and hydrogen. Hydrocarbons can be gases, liquids, or solids. Propane (a gas), octane (a liquid), and wax (a solid) all consist of hydrocarbons.

Hygrometer: An instrument that measures relative humidity.

Hypersensitivity pneumonitis (HP):   A pulmonary disease characterized by inflammation and fibrosis, often caused by an allergic response to inhaling bioaerosols.

Hyphae (sing. hypha):   The rootlike threads of fungi.

IAQ: Indoor air quality.

Immiscible: Not mixable. Two liquids (such as oil and water) that separate into layers are immiscible.

Immunoglobulin: A protein having antibody activity, found in the blood or other body fluids.

Incomplete combustion: Combustion that results in the formation of soot, carbon monoxide, or both. In contrast, when combustion is complete, all carbon is combined with oxygen to form carbon dioxide.

Infiltration: Pressure-driven flow of air into a building or some other defined space; the opposite of exfiltration.

Infrared energy: A form of light energy associated with radiant heat transfer through a vacuum or a gas. Infrared energy can be felt as heat on the skin and can be reflected by a mirror and focused like light, but it cannot be seen except with the aid of a "night scope."

Larva (pl. larvae):   The juvenile form of some insects and animals. The larvae of many insects are wingless and look like small worms. A maggot is a fly larva.

Linseed oil: A nonedible vegetable oil obtained from flaxseed and used as a binder in paint.

Media filter: A pleated filter made from fiberglass that looks like a thick piece of folded paper.

Medium-density fiberboard (MDF):   A composite of wood and formaldehyde-containing glue.

Mesothelioma: A type of chest cancer caused by inhalation of asbestos fibers.

Meter: A unit of measurement equal to about thirty-nine inches.

Methylene chloride: A chlorinated hydrocarbon solvent with a very low boiling point that is a component of many paint strippers.

Microgram.   *See* Gram.

Micron: A measure of length equal to one millionth of a meter, about 0.0004 inch.

Mildew: Fungus (mold) that appears to grow primarily on surfaces.

Milligram.   *See* Gram.

Mites: Tiny members of the arachnid family. Most species live in the soil, but others are associated with animals and insects. Dust mites, found in pillows, mattresses, and carpets, subsist on skin scales and cause asthma symptoms.

Mixture: A combination of materials that can be separated by physical means (such as a strainer or filter).

Moisture meter: A device used to determine the moisture content of wood or other materials.

Mold: A slimy or powdery growth caused by fungi. Molds require oxygen and water to flourish, but they also need a source of nutrients such as wood or other plant materials.

Mold spore: The reproductive cell (or cells) of fungi, usually microscopic and dispersed into the air. Most spores contain allergens, and many contain mycotoxins.

Mud tube: Hollow tubes constructed of sand and termite secretions; also referred to as a shelter tube.

Mycotoxin: A toxin produced by a fungus. Some mycotoxins are carcinogenic, others are immunosuppressants.

Ochratoxin-A: A mycotoxin made by species of *Aspergillus* and *Penicillium*.

Off-gassing: Emission of a solvent or other chemical from the surface of a solid into the air; also referred to as out-gassing.

Oil safety valve (OSV):   A control placed on an oil tank or line that prevents oil from leaking through a punctured oil line when the burner pump is not operating.

Open-cell foam.   *See* Closed-cell foam.

Out-gassing.   *See* Off-gassing.

Ozone (O_3):   An unstable form of oxygen (O_2) formed by electric sparks or ultraviolet light in air.

Panned bay: A return duct that is formed by installing sheet metal between two or more joists.

Particulate: A microscopic fragment of a solid or droplet of a liquid that is suspended in air. Particulates vary in size. If large, they may settle on surfaces; if small, they may remain suspended.

Penicillium: A genus of fungi. Some *Penicillium* produce the antibiotic penicillin; one species, *P. camemberti,* is used to make Camembert cheese.

Phases of matter: States of matter. The three states or phases of matter are solid, liquid, and gas.

Phase change: The changing of a substance from one state of matter to another. Phase changes include freezing and melting, condensation, and boiling and evaporation. During a phase change, a substance is not chemically altered, but its physical properties (or characteristics such as color, density, or conductivity) change.

Pigment: In paint, a powder used to hide or to introduce color. Most pigments are ground-up minerals.

Plenum: Part of the air conveyance system in which the pressure of the air is greater (as in supply ducts) or less (as in return ducts) than that of the outside atmosphere. In office buildings, the space between the suspended ceiling and the floor above serves as a return plenum.

Polyethylene: A solid combustible hydrocarbon "polymer" (a long chain of molecules or atoms) of ethylene that burns with the odor of wax. Most garbage bags are made of polyethylene.

Pressure-treated wood: Wood containing a preservative that permeates much of the wood structure rather than simply coating the surface. Copper arsenate is typically used as the preservative.

Radiant heat: Heat energy that is infrared. All objects, unless they are at absolute zero, radiate heat, which is a form of energy. The hotter something is, the more heat it radiates. If the temperature of an object is high enough (above 1,000°F), light is radiated as well as heat.

Radiation: The emission of energy. There is an entire spectrum (from low to high energy) that includes radio waves, microwaves, infrared, visible light, ultraviolet light, X rays, and gamma rays. Note that nuclear radiation may refer to subatomic particles as well as energy.

Radon: A radioactive cancer-causing gas released from soils containing uranium.

Register: A rectangular device with louvers (slats) at the end of a duct in an air conditioning or a hot-air heating system that spreads out the airflow. A register usually has a damper to control the intensity of the flow.

Relative humidity: A measure of how saturated the air is with moisture at any given temperature or how close the air temperature is to the dew point.

Respirable particle: A suspended particulate under 0.0001 inch (2.5 microns) and therefore small enough to enter deeply into the lungs.

Ridge vent: A simple device installed at the ridge of a roof to cover an opening along the ridge and designed to let air flow out of the attic as well as to prevent rain from wetting the structure. Ridge vents are usually installed in conjunction with soffit vents.

Sill (of a house):   A horizontal piece of framing wood, usually resting on the foundation or other masonry, at the bottom of an exterior wall. The sill is the first piece of wood the wall framing is attached to.

Sleepers: Strips of wood installed on a concrete floor to support the plywood subfloor.

Smoke: Suspended particulates in air that may be either a liquid or solid.

Soffit: The lower enclosed portion of a roof overhang. The soffit consists of a lower horizontal piece (the soffit board) and a long perpendicular attached vertical board (the fascia) that together create the enclosure. The fascia board is nailed to the rafter ends, and a gutter is usually nailed to the fascia.

Soffit vents: Openings in the soffit board that allow air to flow into the soffit to ventilate an attic.

Spore. *See* Mold spore.

Sporulation: The production of spores as a fungus or mold colony matures.

Stachybotrys: A dark brown or black genus of mold that may be associated with sudden infant death syndrome (SIDS). The species *Stachybotrys chartarum* (also known as *S. atra*) produces trichothecene mycotoxins.

Stack pipe: A vertical pipe, three or four inches in diameter, that goes from the basement through the roof (where is it called the plumbing vent). All waste water flows through drain pipes into the stack and from there into the sewer or septic system.

Styrene: An irritating and possibly carcinogenic volatile hydrocarbon used to manufacture the polystyrene plastic found in many products, including computer and television cases and insulating foams.

Sump pump: Typically, a pump that sits in the sump (a hole in the basement floor) to remove water from beneath the floor.

Swale: A depression excavated at the base of a contoured mound of earth, often used to channel water away from a house.

Swamp cooler: A device that uses the evaporation of water to cool air. Swamp coolers are found mainly in the Southwest and function like evaporative pad humidifiers.

Thermal decomposition: A chemical change caused by the addition of heat energy. When food is thermally decomposed, charcoal is produced.

Thoroseal: A portland cement product that is mixed with water and used to seal foundations at the inside.

Treated wood: Wood to which chemicals such as creosote, copper arsenate, and disodium octaborate have been added. These chemicals make the wood resistant to decay caused by bacteria, mold, and insects. *See also Pressure-treated wood.*

Trichothecenes: A series of toxic chemicals (mycotoxins) produced by fungi such as *Stachybotrys chartarum* (common on chronically wet drywall) and *Fusarium graminearum* (common on damp stored corn). The latter fungus produces vomitoxin, a powerful emetic (causing vomiting) for pigs that eat the contaminated corn.

Urea formaldehyde foam insulation (UFFI):   A friable (easily reduced to dust), low-density open-cell foam. UFFI was banned by the U.S. Consumer Product Safety Commission (CPSC) because it off-gassed formaldehyde, a toxic gas that causes illness.

Vadose zone: The zone of soil above the water table where pores in the soil are filled with air and water vapor, not liquid water.

Vapor: The gaseous state of a liquid. Pure steam in a pipe is water vapor, a colorless gas.

Ventilation rate: The amount of fresh air supplied to a space. The ventilation rate is commonly expressed as cubic feet of air per minute (cfm) or air changes per hour (ACH).

Viable: Having the capacity to germinate and grow. Viable spores, under appropriate conditions, lead to fungal growth. Nonviable spores are dead and usually outnumber viable spores in indoor air by a factor of between three and ten to one.

Viscosity: The resistance to flow ("thickness") of a liquid or gas. Water has a low viscosity compared with honey and ketchup.

Water table: The level in the soil below the vadose zone in which all pores in the soil are filled with liquid water rather than air and water vapor.

Water vapor: Water in its gaseous state.

Yeast: Single-celled microscopic organisms, many of which reproduce by budding.

RESOURCE GUIDE

Organizations for Homeowners

- The American Society of Home Inspectors (ASHI) in Des Plaines, Illinois (800-743-2744; http://www.ashi.com), has chapters nationwide and will provide the names of member home inspectors.
- The Association of Indoor Air Quality Investigators (AIAQI), Cambridge, Massachusetts (http://www.AIAQI.org), will provide names of IAQ professionals.
- The U.S. Environmental Protection Agency (EPA) has an indoor air quality home page at http://www.epa.gov/iaq.
- Indoor Air Quality Information Clearing House (800-438-4318) is the EPA's indoor air quality information hotline.
- MyHouseIsKillingMe.com and http://www.jmhi.com provide additional information on IAQ references, products, and services.
- The Institute of Inspection, Cleaning and Restoration Certification (IICRC) (360-693-5675; http://www.iicrc.org) certifies carpet cleaners.

Products and Services for Homeowners

- Envirotech in Cambridge, Massachusetts (617-492-2400; http://www.breatheasier.com), cleans ducts and carries out residential and commercial mold remediation projects.
- Home Environmental in Lexington, Massachusetts (781-862-2873;

http://www.homeenv.com), sells a variety of products for people with allergies and asthma.

- The N95 NIOSH double-strap, fine-particle mask is available in most hardware stores; brands include 3M #8210 and Gerson #1710.

- Neutocrete in Brookfield, Connecticut (888-799-9997; http://www.neutocrete.com), installs a material used to seal dirt floors in crawl spaces.

- The Nisus Corporation in Rockford, Tennessee (800-264-0870; http://www.nisuscorp.com), manufactures Bora-Care and Tim-bor (disodium octaborate tetrahydrate), used to minimize mold and insect infestations. Note that Bora-Care contains ethylene glycol, which can be a problem for people who are chemically sensitive. If in doubt, use Tim-bor. In most states, these products must be professionally applied.

- Research Products Corporation in Madison, Wisconsin (http://www.Aprilaire.com), manufactures the Aprilaire high-efficiency media filter, formerly known as Space-Gard.

- Therma-Stor in Madison, Wisconsin (800-533-7533; http://www.thermastor.com), manufactures the Santa Fe Ultra Efficient Dehumidifier.

- Thoroseal is a water-based portland cement foundation sealant, manufactured by Thoro and available at most building supply outlets.

Products and Services for IAQ Professionals

- Allergenco in San Antonio, Texas (210-822-4116), sells the MK III for air particulate sampling and the invaluable book by E. Grant Smith, *Sampling and Identifying Allergenic Pollens and Molds: An Illustrated Identification Manual for Air Samplers* (San Antonio, Tex.: Blewstone Press, 1990).

- Andersen Instruments in Smyrna, Georgia (800-241-6898), sells instruments for sampling onto petri dishes.

- Bacharach in Pittsburgh, Pennsylvania (800-736-4666), manufactures the Bacharach Monoxor II, an instrument for measuring the concentration of carbon monoxide.

- Burkard Industries in Hertfordshire, England (011-44-1923-773134), manufactures the Personal Volumetric Air Sampler, an instrument for air particulate sampling.

- P&K Microbiology Labs in Cherry Hill, New Jersey (856-427-4044), accepts mold samples from IAQ professionals.
- Professional Equipment in Hauppauge, New York (800-334-9291; http://www.professionalequipment.com), sells the TIF 8800 combustible gas detector and the Tramex moisture meter.
- Romer Labs in Union, Missouri (636-583-8600; http://www.romerlabs.com), tests grains, feeds, and foods for mycotoxins.

Publications

- "Building Air Quality: A Guide for Building Owners and Facility Managers," an EPA publication, available through the Indoor Air Quality Information Clearing House (800-438-4318), or look at http://www.epa.gov/iaq.
- "A Citizen's Guide to Radon," an EPA publication, available through the Indoor Air Quality Information Clearing House (800-438-4318) or look at http://www.epa.gov/iaq.
- "Clean-up Procedures for Mold in Houses," available from the Canadian Mortgage and Housing Corporation (613-748-2367).
- "Cleaning up Your House after a Flood," available from the Canadian Mortgage and Housing Corporation (613-748-2367).
- John Bower, *The Healthy House*, 4th ed. (Bloomington, Ind.: Healthy House Institute, 2001).
- "Indoor Air Quality: Tools for Schools," the EPA's action kit, which offers parents and educators a practical plan for solving IAQ problems in school buildings, available through the Indoor Air Quality Information Clearing House (800-438-4318), or look at http://www.epa.gov/iaq.

INDEX

acaricide powder, 47, 261
acetone, 292
acrolein, 101
actinomycetes, 31; and humidifiers, 57, 180
adhesives: carpet, 303; floor, 39
aflatoxin B$_1$, 18
air, particulates in, 2. *See also* indoor air quality (IAQ); particulates
air conditioners, 61–63, 65; in attics, 221, 224–25, 226; in automobiles, 288; and dehumidifying, 187; filter for, 185; mold associated with, 182–86; odor from, 185, 186; in office buildings, 297–98, 299; overflow tray for, 226, 229; as source of contamination, 182–86, 189. *See also* heating systems
air-drying, 121
air exchange rate, 166, 299–301
airflow, 3, 55; from basements, 125–26, 129–30, 133–34, 137–38; from garages, 283
air handling unit (AHU), 166, 185, 186, 189; in attics, 221, 224–25
air purifiers, 263–64
air quality. *See* indoor air quality (IAQ)

air-to-air heat exchangers, 187, 251–52
Allergenco air sampler, 10, 55
allergens, 4; adhering to airborne particles, 301–3; air conditioners as source of, 61–63, 65; in bedding, 53–55; in clothing, 55, 61, 65, 116; in firewood, 84; fish tanks as source of, 59–60; in furniture, 40–41, 91–92, 94; in hair, 265; in laundry areas, 113–15; plants as, 42–43; soot as, 86–88. *See also* dust; mold
allergies, 1; to animals, 45–46; to food, 105–6; to latex, 302–3; symptoms of, 5, 308, 309–10; yeast, 32
Alternaria fungi, 186
American Society of Home Inspectors (ASHI), 168, 218
ammonia, 107–8, 112, 259, 266
amyl alcohol, 47
anaphylaxis, 136, 212
Andersen air sampler, 138, 169
animals. *See* pets; rodents
animals, stuffed, 22, 60–61
animal urine, 44, 159. *See also* litter boxes; pets
antifreeze, 291
ants, 2, 29–31; in attics, 214